Dr. Cass Ingr[am]

Nutrition
Tests
for
Better
Health

with Judy Kay Gray, M. S.

KNOWLEDGE HOUSE
Buffalo Grove, Illinois

This book was formerly published in 1994 as *The Self Test Nutrition Guide.*
This is a completely revised and expanded addition.

Printed in the United States of America on recycled paper.

First Edition

Disclaimer: This book is not intended as a substitute for medical
diagnosis or treatment. Anyone who has a serious disease should consult a
physician before initiating any change in treatment or before beginning any
new treatment.

ISBN 1-931078-08-4

To order additional copies call 1-800-243-5242 or send an e-mail to
droregano@aol.com. For product or further book information view the
Web site: Oreganol.com
For overseas orders send an e-mail to droregano@aol.com or call
1-847-473-4700.

Table of Contents

Section II - The Dietary Tests

Forward

Nutritional deficiency is a major cause of disease and ill health, even in the Western world. The majority of individuals living in Westernized countries, such as the USA, Canada, Britain, Australia, and Germany, consume a considerable amount of processed food. As a result, nutritional deficiencies are inevitable. In fact, in many instances the deficiencies are extreme. Research proves that common epidemic diseases—heart disease, high blood pressure, diabetes, arthritis, hormonal disorders, cancer, and more—are directly due to nutritional deficiencies. Unfortunately, Americans have been led to believe that they are immune to the occurrence of significant nutritional deficiencies. This belief has been perpetuated largely by the medical profession and dietitians. Simply put, the orthodox belief is that the typical American diet amply supplies an individual's nutritional needs. Yet, this is merely what the medical profession *believes*. The fact is the medical profession has never provided proof for its claims. Research and clinical experience have thoroughly documented the existence of widespread nutritional imbalances and deficiencies in Americans. It is scientifically accepted that a wide range of mental and physical diseases are due exclusively to nutritional deficiencies. Yet, why not? Tens of thousands of research articles are published every year, many in prominent medical journals, proving that *nutritional deficiencies and dietary imbalances play a greater role than any other factor in the cause of ill health.*

Introduction

Wouldn't you like to know where you stand nutritionally? Optimal health is directly dependent upon how well we are nourished. Therefore, the crucial question is: Is the person deficient in specific nutrients, or is he/she getting all the necessary vitamins, minerals, enzymes, fats, proteins, and carbohydrates?

The majority of people would like to learn as much as they can about their nutritional status. Students of nutrition are aware that the potential for achieving optimal health is largely dependent upon the quality of their diets as well as how thoroughly any existing nutritional deficiencies are determined and corrected.

The nutritional status of each person changes rapidly. Each year it changes significantly, even every month, in fact, every day—rather every meal—significant changes occur. These variations are based upon such factors as social habits, medical care (such as drug therapy and/or surgery) exercise (or a lack of it), mental stress, weather conditions, the consumption of or exposure to toxins, and the consumption of refined foods. For instance, an individual who is exercising in hot weather and sweats excessively may rapidly develop a deficiency in sodium and potassium, as well as vitamin C, despite being physically fit, while another person staying indoors in an air conditioned room might have all the vitamin C and sodium he/she needs.

In contrast, an individual living in a cold climate will readily become deficient in pantothenic acid, a nutrient crucial for maintaining the adrenal glands' response to cold weather. A surgical patient's nutritional status might be adequate prior to surgery, but afterwards he/she would likely become deficient in anti-stress nutrients such as vitamin C, pantothenic acid, riboflavin, zinc, selenium, magnesium, and amino acids. An individual taking cortisone readily becomes deficient in vitamin C and calcium, while someone who frequently consumes antibiotics will develop significant B-vitamin deficiencies. A person who eats a candy bar destroys most of his/her chromium and B-vitamin stores, while a person who eats a steak or baked potato, hopefully, with a dusting of a natural concentrate, such as crude red sour grape, adds to them. In other words, whole unprocessed foods provide nutrients, while refined foods destroy them.

Thus, in determining nutritional status it is important to realize that each person's circumstances are different and that there are numerous variables to consider. Additionally, the extent of the nutritional deficits that an individual suffers is often dictated by genetics. For instance, an inherited defect in B-6 metabolism may result in the need for as much as one hundred times the B-6 required by a normal individual.

Stress also determines nutritional requirements. For example, an individual experiencing mental duress, such as grief resulting from the loss of a loved one, marital discord, etc., may require significantly larger amounts of vitamin C, zinc, and/or pantothenic acid compared to a person whose life is relatively stress-free. Pregnant and/or lactating women provide another illustration of the tremendous variation in nutritional requirements. They may require a significantly greater intake of certain nutrients than do women who are not pregnant. However, despite these variables, the majority of individuals desire to know precisely what their nutritional status is so that corrective supplementation, as well as dietary changes, can be prescribed. Yet, most people lack a clear-cut method for making such determinations.

Certainly, it would seem, the medical profession is obligated to apply scientifically based methods for determining nutritional status, since for every disease there is a nutritional component. It is reasonable to presume that in regard to nutritionally induced diseases it is the physician's responsibility to become knowledgeable concerning the symptoms and consequences of nutritional deficiency. This is so the appropriate diagnosis (or diagnoses) can be made. Further, it could be concluded that if an individual is suffering ill health as a result of nutritional deficiencies, his/her physician should be capable of performing various examinations, blood tests, and procedures in order to confirm precisely which nutritional deficiencies he/she has. This is a scientific approach to the diagnosis and treatment of disease. Thus, such an approach would help eliminate the guesswork which is so commonly applied in today's medical scene. Yet, in most medical practices guesswork is the rule. This is because when a patient suffers from nutritional deficiencies physicians possess little knowledge about nutritional diagnosis and know even less about nutritional prescription. Thus, the patient's condition remains undiagnosed, in fact, misdiagnosed.

The complexity of the human body's nutritional chemistry can be compared to a puzzle. Each nutrient is like a piece of the puzzle, and the puzzle is never completed until the status of every nutrient is assessed. What's more, each disease can be regarded as a separate puzzle with its own unique "nutritional topography." Researchers have proven that every major disease has its own pattern of nutritional inadequacies. *It has also been determined that virtually every disease can be improved through diet.* Yet, the vast majority of today's physicians tend to minimize the crucial role played by nutritional deficiencies and/or dietary imbalances in the causation of disease. Physicians often minimize the role of diet in reversing deficiencies. It is as if they have something better to offer—but they don't. Their only alternatives are drugs or similar therapies, which offer little hope for relief or cure.

Today, in America nutritional deficiencies are rampant. True, it is rare to find a fulminant case of scurvy, starvation (i.e. kwashiorkor), or beriberi. However, such extremes of nutritional deficiency represent only a tiny proportion of the innumerable illnesses caused by nutritional deficits. Even so, certain severe nutritional deficiency diseases are far from rare. Rickets, which is due to vitamin D deficiency, is an example of a classical nutritional deficiency disease, and it is increasing in incidence, even here in the United States. Hundreds of thousands of American children are afflicted with it, although black and inner city populations are particularly affected. What's more, strict diets, including vegetarian or vegan diets, may precipitate it. People often make fun of "bow-legged" children and/or teenagers. However, these children most likely have rickets, and no one realizes it.

A number of other serious problems can result from nutritional deficiencies. Each year thousands of Americans are afflicted with a life-threatening disease, which is, in fact, a manifestation of beriberi. It's called *Wernicke-Korsakoff's Psychosis,* and the victims are primarily alcoholics, whose brains are destroyed as a result of alcohol-induced thiamine deficiency. Untold millions of Americans suffer from another potentially life-threatening illness due almost exclusively to vitamin deficiency: pernicious anemia. This disease is the result of a deficiency of vitamin B-12. With this type of anemia there are usually plenty of red blood cells. However, the shape of the cells becomes distorted, and cells actually become enlarged. As a consequence of the genetic defects resulting from B-12 deficiency the oxygen-carrying capacity of the red cells is significantly diminished. This leads to a variety of symptoms, including fatigue, lassitude, headaches, memory loss, depression, and mental confusion.

Perhaps the most common manifestations of pernicious anemia are the neuropsychiatric disorders which are associated with it. B-12 is involved in the synthesis of neurotransmitters, the chemicals which send messages within the brain and along the nerve sheaths. Recent research indicates that a growing body of individuals are developing psychiatric disorders, notably depression, paranoia, psychosis, and dementia, from poor vitamin B-12 nutriture. The elderly are particularly vulnerable, with some studies documenting low blood levels of B-12 in as many as one-third of psychiatric patients over 55.

Thus, pernicious anemia, like scurvy, rickets, pellagra, or beriberi, is mainly a nutritional deficiency disease. In fact, virtually all types of anemia are caused by nutritional deficiency, with iron deficit being the usual missing link, although protein, B-vitamin, and other mineral deficiencies may also play a role.

In contrast, the medical profession primarily recommends drugs for the treatment of diseases, even those caused by nutritional disturbances. Aspirin is one prominent example. There is an intensive media blitz touting the "curative" value of aspirin for a wide range of diseases, including stroke, heart disease, hardening of the arteries, headaches, and even cancer. Lately, this drug has been recommended in medical journals as a prevention for digestive cancer. This recommendation can hardly be taken seriously, since aspirin causes a variety of digestive ailments. Despite this the medical profession continues to aggressively recommend it. It's as if there is a global aspirin deficiency that is responsible for the maladies plaguing modern civilization. Ironically, medical literature supports the fact that aspirin *causes* a greater amount of disease than it cures and is, in fact, responsible for its own unique and potentially fatal disease: *Reye's Syndrome*. Further, several thousand individuals are admitted to hospitals every year in the United States alone as a result of aspirin toxicity; many die.

Aspirin destroys nutrients, including vitamin C, vitamin E, and folic acid. The fact is heart disease and arterial disease—the very diseases aspirin is used for—are caused by a deficiency of these nutrients.

Because of its blood-thinning action and also because it destroys vitamin C, aspirin is the primary cause of acute bleeding from the stomach and/or intestine. Strokes (cerebral hemorrhage) can also result from aspirin consumption, since the blood vessel walls of the brain are weakened by it. In fact, the number of individuals who die every year as a result of aspirin-induced internal bleeding numbers in the thousands.

Aspirin never was and never will be a miracle cure. Those who believe that it is the magic bullet should be aware that for every tablet consumed, the body loses several million molecules of vitamin C, beta carotene, selenium, vitamin E, vitamin K and essential fatty acids, since aspirin aggressively destroys these protective nutrients.

Nutritional deficiency is common in the United States. In some populations it is endemic, and in others it has become a rampant plague. For instance, all alcoholics are nutritionally deficient. Are there not millions of them?

The American public is obviously fraught with illness. In fact, the United States is the most disease-stricken society on earth. Cancer, heart disease, diabetes, stroke, arthritis, lupus, multiple sclerosis, Alzheimer's disease, Parkinson's disease, psoriasis, colitis, hepatitis, obesity, depression, migraine headaches, and an assortment of other degenerative diseases afflict tens of millions. Additional untold millions suffer from vague complaints for which no diagnosis can be determined. These individuals with undetermined deficiencies are on the fringes, wavering between generalized ill health and frank disease. Thus, Americans are taking billions of doses of drugs every year with good reason: they are sick and in pain.

Unfortunately, less than five percent of America's physicians receive training in nutrition. Those who do take nutrition classes gain, at best, a cursory review. Today's physicians lack the skill necessary for diagnosing illnesses caused by nutritional deficiencies and often fail to recognize those caused by gross nutritional deficiency such as beriberi, scurvy, rickets, pernicious anemia, and pellagra. Doctors are simply unaware of the roles played by vitamin, mineral, protein, enzyme, and/or fatty acid deficiencies in the cause of generalized illness as well as gross disease. However, the primary reason for this "medical deficiency" is not merely the doctors' lack of training, it seems that most physicians simply do not believe that poor or inadequate nutrition initiates disease. This is difficult to understand, since the medical journals are replete with data supporting the fact that nutritional deficiencies are a primary cause of chronic ill health. It is also despite the frequent nutrition-related endorsements by the National Cancer Institute, World Health Organization, and numerous other prestigious associations. Recently, the American Medical Association recognized the ineptness of medical professionals regarding nutritional awareness. They noted that the physicians of the future must discipline themselves to spend more time with their patients in the realm of nutritional and/or dietary advice.

Doctors appear to have an attitude problem concerning nutrition. Many feel that making a habit of giving out nutritional advice is beneath them and should be left to the dietitians. They feel that their time should be devoted to "real medicine," that is drug therapy, invasive diagnostics, and surgery. After all, how can dietary intervention compare in curative power to potent drugs? How can improvements in diet and vitamin/mineral therapy rate with high-tech procedures such as laser surgery, angiography, angioplasty, and bypass surgery? How could nutritional medicines and herbal therapies possibly compare with chemotherapy and radiation? Right or wrong, this is how many doctors think today.

The vast majority of medical professionals rely almost exclusively upon drugs and surgical procedures as the basis of treatment. These therapies are often described in medical circles as the "big guns," although they strike more like shotgun blasts than bull's-eye bullets. In contrast, research and clinical experience have proven that nutritional therapy can compare in effectiveness to orthodox medicine. Not only is it less toxic, but it is also often more specific and effective than comparable medical approaches. The recent discovery of the Pacific Yew tree's effectiveness against ovarian cancer has proven that.

The typical nutritional recommendations given by doctors today are appalling to the sophisticated nutritionally-oriented mind. Seeking advice from traditional doctors about nutrition is truly putting one's trust with the ignorant. It's like asking directions from someone who doesn't know the way; you are likely to be steered in the wrong direction. Millions of Americans are advised by physicians and/or dietitians to eat margarine instead of butter, imitation cream instead of real cream, fake eggs instead of real eggs, synthetic cheese instead of real cheese, or artificial ice cream instead of real ice cream, soybeans instead of meat. We are told, "Stay away from avocados. They contain too much fat and cholesterol." Avocados do contain fat, but they have been wrongfully associated with cholesterol; they contain none. This is only one example of the nutritional nonsense continually being parlayed by so-called health authorities.

The low-fat milk theory is equally ludicrous. Americans are instructed to drink only skim milk (or 1 % milk) and eat only skim milk cheese. How could highly processed milk products, as skimmed milk products are, be more health-enhancing than pure unprocessed milk[1] as it exists in nature? The fact is as much as 75% of the vitamins and minerals in milk are found in the fat, and, thus, the process of skimming and adulterating milk destroys much of its nutritional value. Recent research has confirmed that studies conducted at the University of Massachusetts determined that skimmed milk products are detrimental, increasing the risks for cataracts, cancer, and heart disease.

Even though this is precisely the opposite of what the American public is being told about milk products, there is good substance for this alternative view. Milk is a whole food. Processing it by removing its fat disrupts its nutritional value and

---

1. "Pure unprocessed milk" is also referred to in the remainder of this book as "whole milk" or "fresh milk." Dietary recommendations for milk should be interpreted to mean whole unprocessed milk. Unprocessed ideally means milk not pasteurized or homogenized, in other words "raw" milk. Unfortunately, even certified raw milk has been banned in most states. Unhomogenized (but pasteurized) goat's milk is available in numerous farm states, including California, Iowa, Illinois, Minnesota, and Wisconsin.

makes it less digestible. Here is why. Milk naturally contains sugar in the form of lactose. Chemically, lactose is a disaccharide, meaning that it is composed of two sugar molecules bound together by chemical bonds. One of these sugars, galactose, can be highly irritating if separated from the milk sugar bonds. That is precisely why fat naturally occurs in milk. It acts as a sealant, protecting the lactose from being destroyed and, thus, preventing the release of the highly irritating galactose. When the fat is skimmed from the milk, the lactose is vulnerable to oxidation, and this results in the release of free galactose. Apparently, the potential toxicity from the free galactose is such that if enough of it accumulates in the body, tissue damage may result. This at least partially explains the research finding that people who regularly consume skimmed milk products instead of those made with whole milk have as much as a threefold higher risk for certain diseases, notably cancer, hardening of the arteries, cataracts, and heart disease.

Currently, beans are being touted as an exceptional food source. However, they fare poorly as a source of quality nutrition when compared to traditional protein sources such as meats, fish, eggs, and milk products. What's more, bean allergy is common, and the major culprits are kidney beans, pinto beans, and mung beans. Legumes, which are related to the bean family, are a richer source of protein, minerals, and vitamins than beans. Yet, here again, allergy is a significant problem, as tens of millions of Americans are intolerant to the various foods of the legume family, particularly peanuts, lentils, split peas, soy beans, and/or chick peas. However, for those who can tolerate them, legumes are an excellent source of nutrients and are usually preferable to beans. In fact, beans are one of the most indigestible of all foods, because as originally described by Johnathon Wright, M. D. they contain natural chemicals called lectins. These compounds frequently provoke severe allergic intolerances and gastrointestinal distress. Beans cannot be regarded as an adequate replacement for the super-nutrition foods that nutritionists are attempting to displace by them.

Imitation or "laboratory" food is a modern food scheme. Synthetic food is always inferior to real food. There is no nutritional value in coffee creamer: no viable vitamins, fatty acids, or minerals. Instead, its list of ingredients includes corn syrup, hydrogenated vegetable oils, food dyes, sulfites, and MSG. In contrast, real cream contains numerous nutrients and is usually free of additives. The only justifiable reason for replacing real cream with coffee creamer is in the case of butter-fat or milk allergy, and even then it would be more nutritionally sound to leave it out than to add imitation cream. The same is true of ice cream; if you are going to indulge in it, for heaven's sake eat the real thing with the least amount of additives.

Artificial eggs also fail to bring significant nutritional value to the table. After all, what is the nutritional value of food dyes, hydrogenated oils, artificial flavors, and processed egg whites compared to real eggs? Eggs are loaded with nutrients and are one of Nature's richest sources of protein, vitamin A, folic acid, lecithin, riboflavin, vitamin E, biotin, chromium, iron, and, yes, cholesterol. Compare this list of critical nutrients contained in real eggs with the ingredients found in artificial eggs, which are devoid of virtually all of these aforementioned nutrients. In fact, there simply is no comparison. It is truly appalling that such a senseless recommendation as replacing real eggs with egg substitutes could be made despite its glaringly erroneous nature. Yet, millions of Americans continue to follow such advice, literally like so many lambs being herded by their shepherds to slaughter.

A good rule is to always opt for the foods synthesized by Nature over those synthesized by man. Even as noxious as refined sugar is, it is perhaps less damaging to consume it rather than the sugar substitutes, which are nothing more than synthetic chemicals. The human body has the capacity to digest sugar, since it is a naturally occurring substance. This is not so with the artificial sweeteners, such as NutraSweet and saccharin, both of which are produced from petro-chemical waste products. The safety of these sweeteners for human consumption has never been proven. On the contrary, evidence is accumulating that artificial sweeteners are toxic even in relatively small amounts. Saccharin, which is a coal tar derivative, has long been suspected of being a carcinogen and has been linked to the cause of bladder cancer. NutraSweet causes a wide range of symptoms and illnesses, including temporary and/or permanent blindness, nerve disorders, behavioral disorders, digestive disturbances, and migraine headaches in children and adults.

There are a host of other fake foods and synthetic food additives, far more than can be listed in these pages. All are devoid of nutritional value and, in fact, detract from nutritional status by destroying nutrients and/or impairing their absorption. Here are a few examples. Synthetic iron destroys vitamin E, vitamin C, and beta carotene. Brominating agents, such as those used to fumigate fruit and bleach flour, destroy vitamin C, vitamin E, beta carotene, riboflavin, pantothenic acid, potassium, and selenium. Sulfites oxidize vitamin C, molybdenum, riboflavin, and folic acid. Food dyes inactivate vitamin B-6, folic acid, and vitamin C. Ethylene glycol, the main constituent of antifreeze and a relatively common food additive, destroys vitamins A, C, E, and the mineral selenium. The preservatives BHT and BHA destroy vitamins A, C, and E. EDTA, a chelating agent, prevents the absorption of minerals such as zinc, calcium, and magnesium. Pesticides, residues of which are found in virtually all commercial foods, inactivate vitamin C, vitamin E, B-6, digestive enzymes, and selenium. Chlorine inactivates thiamine and destroys vitamins A, C, and E. Chlorine is found in foods packed in water as well as in all municipal water supplies. Fluoride, which is commonly found in most municipal water supplies, destroys vitamins B-1, C, E, and beta carotene and disrupts the function of virtually all human enzymes.

To make matters worse our food, even if fresh and unprocessed, contains less nutrients than ever before in American history. Commercial farming practices are the main culprits. Prior to the turn of the century all foods grown in this country were "organic". This means they were grown on virgin soil without the use of toxic chemicals. In that age the health-giving qualities of food were regarded as more important than economic concerns. In contrast, the primary goal of modern farmers is to achieve a high yield per acre. The nutritional quality of food is rarely if ever an issue. As a result, Americans survive on food which appears to be normal, but in actuality is nutritionally defective.

Over the past 60 years farmers have dumped untold billions of tons of chemicals in the form of fertilizers, pesticides, fungicides, and herbicides onto the soil. This practice has damaged the soil to such a degree that there are far less nutrients in it compared to the original virgin state. Thus, food grown on depleted soil absorbs a reduced amount of nutrients. What's more, agricultural chemicals bind what few minerals are left in the soil, making them unavailable for absorption into the crops. That is one of the major reasons there is a virtual epidemic of trace mineral deficiency in the USA. As a consequence, ill health is on the rise. Mineral deficiency may be manifested by common symptoms, such as fatigue or depression, and will ultimately cause serious and/or life-threatening diseases.

Many farmers are aware of this critical connection between trace minerals and health. The lack of single trace minerals in the soil can cause a significant reduction in crop yield and, in the extreme, may cause crop failure. Animals readily become mineral deficient if they are fed primarily commercially grown crops. In fact, cattle can be so damaged by a lack of certain minerals that they may become crippled or may even drop dead en masse. Newborn animals are particularly vulnerable to sudden death from nutritional deficiency. Symptoms of mineral deficiency in cattle include hoof and mouth disease, arthritis, belly bloating, diarrhea, weight loss, skin eruptions, lung infections, bone deformities, hair loss, infertility, and loss of appetite.

Pesticides and herbicides bind minerals by an action known as chelation, making them unavailable to plants. Commercial fertilizers also bind minerals. Some examples of the adverse effects of farm chemicals on the soil are as follows:

Chemical	Soil Nutrient
Lime	Binds zinc and manganese and impedes copper intake
Nitrogenous fertilizers	Impair copper absorption into plants
Phosphates	Create excess absorption of molybdenum and impair calcium uptake
Potash (potassium)	Causes boron deficiency in plants
Pesticides/herbicides	Impair the absorption of all essential minerals

The importance of this data is emphasized by the fact that 99% of the food grown in the United States is produced on soil fertilized with commercial fertilizers.

Soil erosion has also contributed to a decline in mineral levels. Thus, it is no surprise that researchers have discovered trace mineral deficiencies in the soil of virtually every state in the country. For instance, some 30 states have suboptimal soil zinc levels. Virtually all have reduced magnesium levels. Few if any states have adequate soil levels of selenium, cobalt, and/or copper. Thus, the food is mineral deficient even before it is fumigated, brominated, chlorinated, refined, sweetened, waxed, stored, or cooked. For these reasons virtually every American whose diet consists of commercially available food is deficient in at least one of the trace minerals and usually several of them.

Trace minerals are the essence of life and are of even greater significance than the vitamins. While they are given the designation of "trace," compared to the quantity of vitamins normally found in the body, they are abundant. They are the essence of life, because they modulate cellular function by stimulating and controlling the rate of cellular reactions. It is through the enzymes that minerals exert this effect, since minerals are the spark plugs which catalyze them. Most human enzymes contain a mineral fixed within amino acids. Take zinc, for example. It is an integral component of hundreds of human enzymes. As a result, zinc is essential for the stimulation of millions of enzymatic reactions every fraction of each second. In fact, such a large number of enzymes are zinc dependent that researchers have been unable to fully quantify them. Other minerals heavily involved in enzymatic functions include magnesium, selenium, copper, manganese, molybdenum, and potassium.

The human body thrives on minerals. Unfortunately, Americans eat few mineral-rich foods. Instead they consume large quantities of mineral-depleted foods such as white flour products (including pasta), white rice, refined corn products, refined sugar, commercially grown fresh produce, and canned produce.

The American public is interested in nutrition, and this interest is growing exponentially every year. People are aware that what they eat has a major influence upon how they feel. They are beginning to realize that the traditional American diet isn't all that it is touted to be. They are starting to feel the difference—the improved energy and enhanced well-being that results from eating right.

An insignificant minority of American physicians practice nutritional medicine, that is the treatment of disease with vitamins, minerals, enzymes, herbs, fatty acids, and other natural substances. Thus, perhaps the greatest "deficiency" in America today is that of the nutritional physician. This is an immense problem, since health—and the loss of it—is a complexity, one which should be addressed by professionals, not the public. Yet, most nutritionally-oriented people know that top-notch nutritional physicians are hard to locate. This problem is most extreme in small cities and towns. However, there is a similar shortage in many major cities. Where these nutritional doctors do exist, the population densities are astronomically high. A city the size of Dallas might have five or ten such physicians, while supporting several thousand traditional doctors.

Physicians who use this book find it particularly effective. This is because it can be used as a historical guide for the evaluation of nutritional illness as well as their elimination. However, it was written primarily for lay people, who are convinced of the health-enhancing value of nutrition. It is also written for those who find it difficult to access nutritionally oriented physicians.

Does this mean that this book is a diagnostic manual, that people can read it and determine precisely what illnesses they have? Not at all. It is simply a guidebook to provide clues for what might be wrong, especially regarding nutrition. Only a licensed medical professional can establish a diagnosis: books can't. Diagnostic testing is the primary method for procuring a diagnosis, and obviously this can only be achieved by a licensed physician. Additionally, a thorough history and physical exam are crucial elements for making a diagnosis. This book is an information source which provides an enjoyable method for learning more about your body. Treat it that way, and you will benefit from it. Use it to make a diagnosis, and you could do yourself harm. Diagnoses are made by health professionals. However, this book can help you be more aware of potentially dangerous symptoms as well as your exact nutritional deficiencies. If you are experiencing any symptoms or signs of serious disease, consult your physician.

It is easy to understand why the American public has developed a growing interest in nutritional therapy. Many people have a certain degree of disillusionment with the medical profession. Drug therapy is being questioned by consumers. Millions of people refuse to take medicines, primarily because they are wary of their toxic effects. Surgery is no longer regarded as an absolute cure of choice. Invasive diagnostic testing is often scary, and the side effects are numerous and potentially serious.

The medical profession has failed to find a cure for common degenerative diseases such as heart disease, arthritis, diabetes, lupus, Alzheimer's disease, and/or cancer. Thus, the incidence of these diseases rises every year. However, what may be of greater concern is the fact that certain diseases previously regarded as rare are dramatically rising in occurrence. The connective tissue diseases are one example. These diseases include lupus, fibromyalgia, fibromyositis, dermatomyositis, scleroderma, rheumatoid arthritis, and osteoarthritis. Nutritional therapy can produce significant improvement in these diseases and, certainly, is of greater value than the drugs currently used to treat them.

Perhaps of greatest concern is the rising incidence of infectious diseases. Children are besieged by episodes of upper respiratory, intestinal, and ear infections. Adults suffer with bouts of colds, flu, food poisoning, kidney/bladder infections, and/or intestinal infections as well as pneumonia. The sexually transmitted diseases are no longer simply a source of embarrassment or chronic illness; they are outright killers and will soon be listed among the top five causes of death in this country. A frightening and recent development is the outbreak of drug-resistant tuberculosis infections. Tuberculosis is also on the rise in children, despite immunizations. This is largely because of outbreaks of drug-resistant strains of TB in hospitals. Furthermore, recent outbreaks have been traced to sites which place untold millions at risk: the air systems/filters in jet airliners. In fact, the circumstance is so ominous that researchers claim all of the advances made in TB treatment over the past century will be reversed in a mere twenty years or less. An additional concern is the Chronic Fatigue Syndrome, a disease which primarily affects adults. This debilitating condition has been correlated to infections by viruses and parasites, although the exact cause remains unknown.

How to Get the Most Out of this Book

The purpose of this book is to educate individuals about nutrition, that is their own personal nutrition. Particular emphasis is placed upon the determination of each individual's nutritional status. At the end of each exam information regarding corrective nutritional supplementation and dietary advice is provided. Those who are willing to change dietary and social habits that impair good nutrition will receive the greatest benefits from this book.

Millions of Americans are "addicted" to certain foods and find the thought of change overwhelming. The fact is the American diet is permeated with addictive substances; caffeine, MSG, sugar, white flour, cocoa, vanilla bean, food dyes, artificial sweeteners, and alcohol are prominent examples. It is not surprising that many Americans find themselves so attached to their dietary and social habits that they feel helplessly and hopelessly addicted. This is certainly true of the majority of coffee, chocolate, cigarette, sugar, and alcohol "junkies." Yet, despite this dilemma, habit restructuring is as simple as this: you can change—*if you want to.*

Heredity and environmental factors play critical roles in influencing the capacity for individuals to readily alter nutritional habits. Family members often share deficiencies. This may be due to genetics, but it may also be the result of environmental factors. Parents who smoke are constantly polluting their children's lungs with cigarette smoke. Not only does the smoke cause nutritional depletion, but it also increases the youths' risks for a variety of diseases, including heart disease, cancer, lung disease, asthma, and immune deficiency. What's more, many children inherit the pattern of deficiencies seen in smokers as a consequence of being exposed to the residues of cigarette smoke while they are in the womb or during their formative years.

Children have little choice but to adhere to the dietary norms of their parents and grandparents. If the parents and/or grandparents are sugar addicts, so too will the children become addicted. However, as bizarre as it may seem, some parents carefully watch their diets while they feed their children all manner of junk food ranging from hot dogs, hamburgers and french fries to Twinkies. Here is the point: all family members should take the quizzes. See if a pattern develops. Then, the entire family can follow a nutritional rebuilding program. It is much easier to adhere to new dietary habits if everyone joins together in the effort.

When taking the tests, a question may arise regarding the past or present: Which is most important as far as analyzing the results? The score that you register right now, which is representative of your current lifestyle, is the most meaningful one. However, it is also of value to test how you would have scored previously, for instance, as a child, teenager, or perhaps as you lived five or ten years ago. This will provide the most comprehensive picture of your nutritional status and will help determine the extent of your nutritional needs.

Family members should assist each other in the disciplinary action required for changing from a processed and junk food diet to the consumption of nutrient-rich whole foods. In other words, they should work together as a team. Inevitably, temptations will overcome discipline, and some people will falter. Encourage such individuals to give it his or her best effort. The benefits from eating right are immense and well worth the endeavor. Better health, improved energy, increased vigor, improved appearance, healthier skin, disease prevention, and, in some instances, the stalling of the aging process are all likely consequences of the effort to eat right.

How to use the tests

In order to evaluate your progress document your symptoms, past and present, in a loose-leaf notebook. Make sure you record the date of the entry and label each group of symptoms under the nutrient deficiency category. The following entries from a typical symptom log is based upon the upcoming vitamin B-1 deficiency test. Obviously, in this example the individual's symptoms have improved:

Date	Symptoms — B1
08/12/93 (first testing)	2. nervousness 7. chronic constipation 13. irritability 39. noise sensitivity 45. insomnia
11/12/93 (note the improvements)	7. constipation (occasional) 13. irritability (rare) 39. noise sensitivity (mild)

After you make dietary improvements and take the appropriate nutritional supplements, it is wise to retest yourself to see if the symptoms have diminished. Do this at least every three months until your symptoms are reduced to your satisfaction. Then check your status periodically—once or twice a year—to maintain a general awareness of your nutritional well-being. Remember, good health is your greatest treasure.

Nutritional tests on the Web: NutritionTest.com.

For many people taking the tests in the book may seem cumbersome. What's more, some people don't like writing out the symptoms. Plus, reading an entire book is time-consuming. Therefore, there is a need for a simplified and fast way to take the tests. Plus, what if the tests must be repeated, which should be done after therapy is applied? It is more difficult to do this and retain the information. This is the benefit of taking the tests on the internet. Nutritiontest.com is the answer. In a mere two hours all the tests may be taken: 46, in total with recommendations included.

The internet is a convenient method to quickly perform the tests. It includes several tests not found in the book. Plus, many of the tests are more extensive than those found in the book.

Nutritional deficiency is an epidemic. Nutritional textbooks make one fact quite clear: that all Americans are deficient. What's more, all children are also deficient. This is merely the consequence of eating depleted food. Nutritiontest.com is the quickest and easiest way to perform the tests and, therefore, to find out exactly what you are deficient in. Use it as an adjunct to this book. The book contains information not found on the site. So, for those who wish the most systematic approach the two work together as a team.

This is a highly thorough system. It will help the individual determine exactly their nutritional imbalances. Plus, it describes how to correct them through food and nutritional supplements. For further information or to sign up for the tests call 1-800-243-5242 (or if overseas call 1-847-473-4700), or send an e-mail to: droregano@hotmail.com. Book owners receive a special discount.

Tests available at Nutritiontest.com are:

Nutrition tests

Vitamins - fat soluble
- Vitamin A
- Vitamin D
- Vitamin E
- Vitamin K

Vitamins - water soluble
- Biotin
- Folic Acid
- Niacin
- Pantothenic acid
- Pyridoxine
- Riboflavin
- Thiamine
- Vitamin B-12
- Vitamin C

Proteins and amino acids
- Digestive enzymes
- Tryptophan

Minerals
- Calcium
- Chromium
- Iodine
- Iron
- Magnesium
- Manganese
- Phosphorus
- Potassium
- Selenium
- Zinc

Specialized nutrients
- Carnitine
- Coenzyme Q-10
- Genetic material (DNA/RNA)
- Taurine
- Water

Antioxidants and Flavonoids
- Beta carotene
- Bioflavonoids
- Glutathione (peroxidase)

Essential fatty acids and lipids
- Essential fatty acids
- Phospholipids

Syndromes
- Adrenal collapse
- Chronic viral infestation
- Estrogen imbalance
- Intestinal parasite
- Lead intoxication
- Liver dysfunction
- Male hormone imbalance
- Mercury intoxication
- Pesticide/herbicide intoxication
- Sluggish thyroid
- Yeast/Fungus infestation

Section I

The
Nutritional
Deficiency Tests

Vitamin B-1 (Thiamine)

The existence of B-vitamins was first conceived less than 100 years ago. In the early 1900s Casimir Funk, a Polish biochemist, proposed the existence of certain dietary substances required in trace amounts for the prevention of diseases that were the plague of that era, notably beriberi and pellagra. Researchers later (1915) determined that food contained both water and fat soluble vitamins. Using egg yolks as the raw material they extracted the vitamins and named the fatty fraction "fat soluble A" and coined the name for the water fraction, "water soluble B". Eventually, chemists were able to isolate two of the vitamins, thiamine and riboflavin, from the water soluble fractions. Once isolated, the chemical formulas of the individual vitamins were identified, and, ultimately, they were synthesized.

However, to their surprise researchers found something highly intriguing. The purified and/or synthetic compounds were considerably less effective than the original crude extracts made from foods. Apparently, a number of other unknown factors worked in concert with the known vitamins. The chemists' intensive search for these unknown factors led to the discovery of the remaining B-vitamins: niacin, folic acid, vitamin B-12, biotin, pantothenic acid, and pyridoxine. Future research will likely reveal yet-to-be-discovered fractions.

Thiamine deficiency is common in the United States. This is despite the fortification of processed foods, notably breads and cereals, with the nutrient. Gross deficiency of thiamine causes a condition known as *polyneuritis*. This is defined as inflammation of the nerve sheaths throughout the body. Obviously, thiamine is required for the normal functioning of the nerves. It is no surprise that this important B-vitamin is known as the *morale vitamin*. In fact, mood changes, depression, and/or other mental symptoms are early signs of its deficiency.

Anyone who believes that thiamine deficiency in America is rare should consider the following study. Volunteers were placed on a standard American menu of bread, processed cereals, well-done beef, potatoes, white rice, gelatin, egg whites, sugar, cocoa, skimmed milk products, canned fruits, canned vegetables, and coffee. The diet was supplemented with every nutrient except thiamine. In addition, the volunteers were given thiamine-deficient brewer's yeast. This was done to ensure that any symptoms that might occur could be assigned exclusively to thiamine deficiency. In fact, the diet was so well supplemented that in all respects, with the exception of thiamine nutriture, it was superior to that eaten by the majority of Americans. According to the researchers, "All the volunteers became irritable, depressed, quarrelsome, uncooperative and... fearful that some misfortune awaited them. Two became so agitated that they felt life was no longer worth living and threatened suicide. In part, this could be attributed to weakness, in part to inability to concentrate, confusion, and uncertainty of memory..."

There are a number of reasons that thiamine deficiency is common in America and other civilized societies. First, the so-called civilized diet is largely composed of highly processed and refined foods, while thiamine occurs naturally in large quantities only in wholesome unprocessed foods. Such foods include whole grains, particularly the germ and bran fractions, fresh organ meats, peanuts, eggs, and soybeans. Secondly, naturally occurring thiamine is a rather delicate compound and is readily destroyed by cooking. Losses during storage may also be significant and fluorescent light negatively affects it. What's more, thiamine is inactivated by chlorine, and, thus, people who wash and/or cook their food with chlorinated water or, more importantly, drink, bathe, or swim in chlorinated water are likely to become thiamine deficient.

One way to prevent thiamine loss while cooking is to add acidic substances, such as lemon juice or vinegar, to the cooking medium. Apparently, acids stabilize the thiamine molecule, preventing heat-induced destruction. Thus, thiamine depletion is reduced when preparing recipes naturally high in acid such as spaghetti sauce, tomato soup, and fish in lemon sauce.

Thiamine is absorbed chiefly from the upper part of the small intestine, i.e. the duodenum. Thus, diseases of that region, for instance, duodenal ulcer, pancreatitis, and giardiasis (a parasitic infestation of the small bowel), greatly hamper thiamine absorption and lead to its deficiency.

People who regularly drink black tea often develop thiamine deficiency, since tea contains compounds which block thiamine absorption. Raw sea foods, such as sushi, herring, oysters, and lox, can induce the deficiency, since these foods contain a thiamine antagonist called thiaminase. In actuality, this is an enzyme which attacks the thiamine molecules, splitting them in half. Individuals who suffer from liver disease of any type (hepatitis, cirrhosis of the liver, Gilbert's disease) are vulnerable for developing severe thiamine deficiency. Additionally, alcohol destroys thiamine. One or more drinks per day is enough to induce a severe deficiency. For chronic alcoholics, particularly those who drink a pint or more of alcohol daily, thiamine deficiency can become so extreme as to result in irreparable nerve and brain damage. The function of all brain cells is thiamine dependent; it is no wonder that thiamine-deficient alcoholics develop a wide range of mental symptoms, including depression, memory loss, agitation, violent behavior, and frank psychosis.

To perform the thiamine test and all subsequent tests, add the total number of positive responses and match your score with the mild, moderate, severe, or extreme deficiency categories. Each response is worth one point unless otherwise indicated. It is desirable to keep a record of your deficiencies and check to see if the symptoms decrease with dietary intervention and supplementation.

THIAMINE TEST (each response worth 1 point)

Which of these apply to you?

1. depression and/or anxiety
2. nervousness
3. sugar intolerance
4. lack of appetite or excessive appetite
5. vague chest pains and/or shortness of breath
6. irregular heartbeat
7. chronic constipation
8. indigestion
9. intolerance to protein-rich foods such as meats, soy beans, milk products, and fish
10. leg cramps after exercising
11. agitation
12. chronic fatigue
13. irritability
14. sleep apnea
15. anger
16. fears and/or paranoia
17. excessively rapid heartbeat with mild or moderate exercise
18. rapid resting heartbeat (80 beats or greater per minute)
19. heaviness and/or weakness of the arms or legs
20. burning and/or numbness of the arms, hands, feet, and/or toes
21. personality changes
22. heartburn
23. swelling of the extremities
24. bloating after eating
25. stomach aches and/or pain
26. attention deficit (i.e. short attention span)
27. mental dullness and/or poor concentration
28. loss of strength

29. vulnerability to insect bites, particularly fleas and mosquitoes
30. bed wetting
31. temper tantrums and/or violent behavior
√ 32. craving for sugar and/or other sweets
33. apathy or feeling of impending doom
34. eye fibrillations (twitches)
35. lack of sensation for urination (lack of urination)
36. loss of muscle tissue in hands and/or legs
37. premenstrual depression
38. painful menses
√ 39. noise sensitivity
40. rapidly aging skin
41. nausea and/or vomiting
√ 42. cold hands, ears, and feet
43. hypotension (low blood pressure)
44. headache
45. insomnia
46. excessive sweating
47. abdominal pain
48. inability to maintain weight
49. foot and wrist drop
50. tendency to stumble while walking or climbing stairs
51. clumsiness
52. sleep walking
53. nightmares
54. chronic swelling of the lymph nodes
55. Do you have an abnormally slow heart rate?
56. Do you have a history of retinal bleeding?
57. Do you have a history of bulimia?
58. Do you regularly consume alcoholic beverages (one or more drinks per day)?
✓ 59. Do you consume black or iced tea on a daily basis?
60. Do you consume raw fish on a daily or weekly basis?
61. Do you have chronic backaches which are unresponsive to traditional therapies?

62. Do you drink two or more cups of coffee on a daily basis?
63. Are you emotionally unstable?
64. Are you quarrelsome or argumentative?
65. Do you have a low pain tolerance?
√ 66. Do you have a phobia of the sensation of creatures (insects) crawling on your skin?
67. Do you have an enlarged heart (cardiomyopathy)?
68. Have you had a portion of your stomach or intestines removed, or have you undergone stomach stapling?
√ 69. Do you adhere to a high carbohydrate diet?

Your Score _____

1 to 9 points *Mild thiamine deficiency:* Even mild thiamine deficiency can result in significant symptoms and predispose individuals to certain diseases. Correct this by eating thiamine-rich foods (see Appendix A) and supplementing the diet with natural thiamine, for instance, Nutri-Sense, which is one of the richest food sources known. Nutri-Sense is a natural thiamine/niacin-rich drink mix made with rice bran and rice polishings, both of which are super-rich in these vitamins. Consume 2 heaping tablespoons of rice polishings-rich Nutri-Sense mixed in milk, water, or juice daily. Additionally, alcohol and refined sugar destroy thiamine, so their intake must be reduced or eliminated.

10 to 21 points *Moderate thiamine deficiency:* Aggressive correction of moderate thiamine deficiency will help prevent future health problems or resolve existing ones, since chronic thiamine deficit often results in a variety of physical and mental derangements. Eat large helpings of thiamine-rich foods and consume 2 to 3 heaping tablespoons of Nutri-Sense twice daily. Additionally, take a multiple vitamin containing thiamine or even better, take fat-soluble thiamine, one or two capsules daily.

Avoid the thiamine destroyers, a category which includes raw fish, green or black tea, coffee, refined sugar, chlorinated water, and alcohol. As a source of easy-to-absorb thiamine eat organic eggs, two to four daily.

22 to 33 points *Severe thiamine deficiency*: A variety of potentially serious medical conditions may result from pro-longed thiamine deficiency. These conditions include malabsorption, underactive or overactive thyroid, dementia, depression, anxiety, congestive heart failure, immune defects, heart rhythm disturbances, hypoglycemia and/or diabetes, and even beriberi. If you have any of these diseases, it is likely that you are thiamine deficient. Correct this deficiency by fortifying baked goods and cereals with Nutri-Sense. In addition, take 3 heaping tablespoons of Nutri-Sense three times daily mixed in juice, water, or milk. Thiamine supplements are also indicated. However, the typical type of thiamine found in vitamin pills, thiamine hydrochloride, is poorly absorbed. Fat-soluble thiamine is a superior type. Take 100 mg (i.e. mg = one milligram = 0.001 gram) of fat-soluble thiamine morning and night. As a source of easy-to-absorb thiamine eat organic eggs, three to four daily. Also, eat organic liver, one serving twice weekly.

34 and above *Extreme thiamine deficiency*: Warning—physiological derangement, as well as internal organ damage, is imminent if tissue thiamine levels continue to decline. The nervous system, including the brain, is particularly vulnerable and can be damaged irreparably unless the deficiency is corrected promptly. Take fat-soluble thiamine, a highly absorbable form of thiamine. The initial dosage should be 300 mg three times daily. After 60 days of this therapy reduce the dosage to 200 mg three times daily. Also, as a source of easy-to-absorb thiamine eat organic eggs, four or more daily. Additionally, fortify foods and cereals with rice bran and/or polishings and mix 4 heaping tablespoons of Nutri-Sense in juice, water, or milk, and drink this mixture morning, noon, and night. If symptoms persist, see your doctor. Also, eat organic liver, one serving three times weekly.

Severe thiamine deficiency can be corrected by injections of this B-vitamin. However, there is a word of caution: intravenous/intramuscular thiamine has been associated with toxicity, including severe allergic reactions. Thus, taking thiamine orally is safer than injections. In fact, evidence is accumulating that the fat-soluble thiamine is the safest form of all. Additionally, it is more readily assimilated. A study was recently performed comparing the absorption of oral doses of fat-soluble thiamine with the absorption of injectable thiamine. The researchers were amazed to find the blood levels were consistently higher with the oral dosage of fat soluble thiamine than with the injectable form.

With the exception of alcoholics suffering from delirium tremens, correction of the thiamine deficiency with oral doses should suffice. For the alcoholic with extreme thiamine deficiency, the next drink might be the fatal one, since life-threatening cardiac and/or neurological symptoms may develop as a result of alcohol-induced thiamine deficiency. Thus, alcoholics who score high on this exam must stop drinking alcoholic beverages immediately. However, they should do so only while under a doctor's care to avoid the delirium tremens, which is potentially fatal. Note: Fat-soluble thiamine and Nutri-Sense drink mix may be purchased from health food stores or by calling 1-800-243-5242.

Vitamin B-2 (Riboflavin)

As early as the 19th century scientists noticed that certain foods possessed a yellow-green fluorescent pigment. They found this pigment in a wide range of foods, including milk, eggs, almonds, organ meats, and vegetables. Because of their fluorescent nature, these pigments were called "flavins", which ultimately led to the naming of riboflavin. Originally, this B-vitamin was called "lactoflavin", since its presence was first observed in milk.

Riboflavin deficiency may be induced by poor nutrition, high consumption of sugar, severe infections, surgery, birth control pills, and/or malabsorption. Other factors which may create a deficiency include lack of stomach acid, antibiotic usage, diuretics, and mental stress. Additionally, malabsorption, high protein intake, faulty lipid metabolism, acute injuries, pregnancy, and lactation all increase the need for riboflavin. The riboflavin content of foods is dependent upon a variety of factors. Farm fresh (unheated, unprocessed) foods offer the highest amounts. Riboflavin losses may be as high as 90% in commercial foods, including "fresh" produce. That is because riboflavin is a highly unstable substance. It is readily destroyed by light, particularly fluorescent light. For example, milk stored in plastic jugs and glass containers loses the majority of its riboflavin content by the time it is consumed.

One of riboflavin's most critical functions relates to oxygen metabolism. Riboflavin accelerates the capacity of the lungs to remove oxygen from the air. In addition, it aids in the transfer of blood oxygen into the cells and is also crucial for the utilization of oxygen at the cellular level. Sufficient riboflavin in the lungs helps protect the body from the ill effects of air pollution.

Top sources of riboflavin include organ meats, muscle meats, eggs, almonds, whole organic milk, whole (organic) milk cheese, caviar and, to a lesser degree, dark green leafy vegetables. Starchy foods, such as beans, grains, and potatoes, are generally poor sources of this vitamin. Additionally, riboflavin is more readily absorbed from meat than from vegetable sources. Riboflavin may well be one of the most difficult of all vitamins to procure in the diet because of its instability and rarity in the food supply.

VITAMIN B-2 (RIBOFLAVIN) TEST
(each response worth 1 point)

Which of these apply to you?

1. inflamed and/or swollen tongue
2. bloodshot eyes or conjunctivitis
3. cracks at the corners of the mouth
4. depression
5. dizziness
6. burning and/or itching of the eyes
7. blurred vision
8. sensitivity of the eyes to light (photophobia)
9. eczema
10. lips which are constantly chapped
11. cholesterol and/or whitehead-like deposits on the face
12. crusting of the eyelids (granulated eyelids)
13. wrinkles radiating from lips towards nose and cheeks
14. poor wound healing
15. excessive tearing of the eyes
16. insomnia
17. unusually red or whitish lips
18. decreased hand grip strength
19. digestive disturbances
20. mood swings
21. nervousness
22. abnormal or excessive appetite
23. a feeling of "sand" under the eyelids
24. chronic acne
25. loss in the width (fullness) of the upper lip
26. fatigue
27. sores around and/or in the mouth
28. lack of concentration
29. irritable colon
30. dandruff

31. painful tongue
32. eye fatigue
33. chronic sinus problems
34. eyelid spasms/twitching
35. myopia (nearsightedness)
36. greasy facial skin, especially on the nose
37. lips which are swollen, inflamed, and/or crack easily
38. scaly greasy lesions on scrotum or vulva
39. tendency to walk or stand with feet turned inward
40. visible tiny red blood vessels about the nose or on the cheeks
41. tongue which is cherry red or reddish blue in color
42. roughening or thickening of the skin on the nose
43. Do you use chewing tobacco?
44. Do you smoke cigarettes (1/2 pack or more per day)?
45. Do you consume alcohol on a regular basis?
46. Do you take birth control pills, or have you in the past taken birth control pills for a prolonged time (five or more years)?
47. Do you suffer from chronic lung disease?
48. Do you urinate frequently or with excessive volume?
49. Have you had your duodenum removed, or are you suffering from duodenal ulcer?
50. Are you taking cholesterol-lowering medications?
51. Do you suffer from retinal detachment or retinitis?
52. Do you have macular degeneration?
53. Do you suffer from corneal ulcers?
54. Do you consume refined sugars on a daily or weekly basis?
55. Do you have chronic dermatitis and/or dermatitis due to light or metal sensitivity?
56. Are you a vegetarian?
57. Do you regularly take diuretics?
58. Do you take antibiotics on a daily, weekly, or monthly basis?
59. Do you have a history of cataracts?
60. Do you have anemia that has failed to respond to iron therapy?

61. Do you sunburn easily, or do you develop rashes from sun exposure?
62. Are you constantly rubbing your eyes?
63. Do you have bald spots (atrophy) on your tongue?

Your Score _____

1 to 8 points *Mild riboflavin deficiency*: Riboflavin is a tightly controlled nutrient in terms of tissue storage/losses, since it is firmly bound within the cells. However, even a modest reduction in tissue stores results in cellular dysfunction. Mild riboflavin deficiency may be corrected by taking a multiple vitamin containing riboflavin and by curtailing the consumption of refined sugar and alcohol, both of which destroy this nutrient. Add hefty portions of riboflavin-rich foods to the diet. Eat organic liver and eggs on a weekly basis; have at least 6 eggs weekly. Food sources of this vitamin are of greater value versus the synthetic. Royal jelly is also an excellent source. A crude unprocessed royal jelly may be taken as capsules. Take Royal Kick, 2 to 4 capsules daily.

9 to 20 points *Moderate riboflavin deficiency*: At this stage individuals may suffer from certain medical conditions, including myopia, astigmatism, alopecia, and/or growth impairment. Correct the deficiency by taking a multiple vitamin containing riboflavin, plus a B-complex tablet containing 25 or 50 mg of riboflavin. Additionally, include riboflavin-rich foods such as organic meats (especially liver), lean red meat, eggs, whole milk products, and fresh dark green leafy vegetables. Eat organic liver and eggs on a weekly basis. Eat at least 10 eggs weekly, that is until the deficiency is corrected. The best vegetable source of riboflavin is the wild green powerdrops: take 4 dropperfuls daily (to order call 1-800-243-5242).

21 to 34 points *Severe riboflavin deficiency:* At this level of deficiency significant impairment of the function of the cells and internal organs develops, especially the liver. An aggressive program should be instituted for replenishing tissue riboflavin stores. Create riboflavin-rich menus. In addition to a multiple vitamin, take a B-complex tablet containing at least 50 mg of riboflavin twice daily. Take also desiccated buffalo liver (4 capsules three times daily), one of the richest natural sources of riboflavin. Strictly avoid refined sugar and alcohol. Eat organic eggs, and drink organic milk on a daily basis. As a natural source of vegetable-based riboflavin take wild green powerdrops, six dropperfuls daily. This product is only available via mail order: 1-800-243-5242.

35 and above *Extreme riboflavin deficiency:* If the tissue riboflavin content falls to a critical level, the system responsible for the production of cellular energy fails to function properly. Furthermore, prolonged, extreme riboflavin deficiency may result in permanent damage of the skin, nerves, and/or internal organs. The skin, hair, and eyes are particularly vulnerable. Diseases such as cataracts, macular degeneration, retinal detachment, eczema, alopecia, and premature aging are likely to occur. One prominant symptom is the reduction in the size of the upper lip. Correct the deficiency by taking 100 mg of riboflavin morning and night. Additionally, take 6 capsules of desiccated buffalo liver 3 times daily. Also take a multiple vitamin containing all the B-vitamins and load up on riboflavin-rich foods, especially organic liver, eggs, and whole milk products. As a natural source of vegetable-based riboflavin take wild green powerdrops, eight or more dropperfuls daily. This product is only available via mail order: 1-800-243-5242.

Vitamin B-3 (Niacin)

The need for niacin was first established as a consequence of the discovery of a severe disease. This disease, called pellagra or "rough skin", was originally described during the 18th century by a Spanish physician. Pellagra was well known to American physicians of the early 20th century, since it was one of the leading causes of illness and death. However, pellagra was unique compared to most of the diseases of that era. It is exclusively a disease of poor diet, the consequence of the refinement of whole grains, corn, and rice. Pellagra is a sort of final proof, however crude and destructive, that "man cannot live on bread alone"—white bread, that is.

Niacin is readily absorbed throughout most of the small intestine. However, mental stress, alcohol/drug abuse, prescription drugs, and processed foods all cause the depletion of this vitamin. Since little niacin is stored in the body, a deficiency may readily occur. As a result, tissue levels must be continually replenished.

Niacin is essential for fat metabolism, transport, and digestion. It helps mobilize fat from adipose tissue, so that it can be burned as energy. It prevents the buildup of cholesterol within the liver and arteries and, thus, is a natural cholesterol-lowering agent. Niacin is also involved in the synthesis of the protective fatty covering of the nerves, the myelin sheath.

Niacin exists in nature in several forms. The most well researched are nicotic acid and niacinamide. The amino acid tryptophan may be regarded as a form of niacin. This is because if niacin stores are depleted, tryptophan is readily converted into it. Thus, a diet rich in tryptophan may provide sufficient niacin, even though the diet is low in the actual vitamin. This is why corn-rich diets induce niacin deficiency, since corn is low in both niacin and tryptophan. Additionally, small amounts of niacin are synthesized in the intestines by normal bacteria flora. Top sources of tryptophan include red meats, poultry, fish, rabbit, cheese, eggs, and sesame seeds. Excellent sources of niacin include organ meats, fresh muscle meats, rice polishings, eggs, and cheeses. Vegetation is relatively low in this vitamin.

VITAMIN B-3 (NIACIN) TEST

Which of these apply to you?

1. lack of appetite
2. muscular weakness
3. indigestion
4. loss of memory and/or mental acuity
5. depression
6. patches of dry scaly skin (rough skin)
7. chronic diarrhea
8. chronic fatigue
9. bad breath
10. emotional instability
11. insomnia
12. chronic headaches
13. vague abdominal pains
14. dementia/senility
15. dermatitis, especially of hands and/or face
16. sore tongue and/or mouth
17. rectal irritation
18. irritability and/or anxiety
19. psychotic behavior
20. mood swings
21. chronic joint pain and stiffness (arthritis)
22. black coloration of the tongue
23. rough patches of skin in the mouth
24. large brown blotches on the skin
25. Do you consume, on average, one or more alcoholic beverages per day?
26. Is your cholesterol level greater than 230 (untreated)?
27. Do you have a history of cocaine, crack, or heroin abuse?
28. Do you have a history of manic-depressive syndrome or schizophrenia?
29. Do you consume refined sugar on a daily or weekly basis?

30. Do you have a duodenal ulcer, or have you had your duodenum removed?
31. Do you consume corn as a major part of your diet (Mexicans, vegetarians, etc.)?
32. Do you have low stomach acid (hypochlorhydria)?
33. Do you have undigested food in the stool?
34. Do you have neurological disease manifested by a loss of sensation, nerve inflammation, and/or nerve damage?
35. Do you have bald spots on the tongue?
36. Do you have deep fissures (trenches) in the tongue?
37. Do you have dermatitis/inflammation of the scrotum?

Your Score ____

---

1 to 6 points *Mild niacin deficiency:* Mental disturbances, such as depression and memory loss, are the most likely consequences of mild niacin deficiency. Fatigue is also a common symptom. Correct this by taking a multiple vitamin tablet containing niacin and by consuming niacin-rich foods, particularly brown rice, tuna, trout, salmon, halibut, peanut butter, poultry, and liver. Additionally, take 2 heaping tablespoons of Nutri-Sense daily.

7 to 14 points *Moderate niacin deficiency:* This degree of niacin deficiency is usually the consequence of a high sugar diet. Refined grains and alcohol are other major niacin destroyers. Niacin is of crucial importance in energy metabolism. Without it, the body's fuels—sugars, starches, and fats—cannot be utilized by the cells, that is burned as fuel. The result is the accumulation of sugars and/or fats within the blood stream. This is the reason that niacin has been utilized as a heart drug. In pharmaceutical dosages it helps reduce abnormally high blood levels of cholesterol and triglycerides. To correct the niacin deficit take a B-complex tablet containing niacin twice daily. Additionally, consume 3 heaping tablespoons of Nutri-Sense twice daily. Supplement the diet with niacin-rich foods, and avoid refined sugars, white flour, refined corn products, white rice, and alcohol. Regarding the latter alcohol rapidly destroys niacin. Strictly avoid it.

15 to 21 points *Severe niacin deficiency*: Warning—severe niacin deficiency is associated with an increased incidence of a variety of diseases, including high cholesterol, diabetes, heart disease, dementia, hypertension, arteriosclerosis, and arthritis. To correct this deficit take a B-complex capsule or tablet morning and night along with 250 mg of niacin. In addition, take 4 to 6 heaping table-spoons of Nutri-Sense three or four times daily and consume hefty helpings of niacin-rich foods. Strictly avoid all alcoholic beverages and refined sugars. Alcohol is a primary cause of niacin deficien-cy. Continuous drinking may result in catastrophic damage to internal organs, specifically as a result of niacin deficiency.

Note: All glandular sources must be organic.

23 and above *Extreme niacin deficiency*: Warning—extreme-niacin deficiency is associated with an increased incidence of a variety of diseases, including high cholesterol, diabetes, heart dis-ease, dementia, hypertension, arteriosclerosis, and arthritis. To correct this deficit take a B-complex capsule or tablet morning and night along with 250 mg of niacin. In addition, take 4 to 6 heaping tablespoons of Nutri-Sense three or four times daily, and consume hefty helpings of niacin-rich foods. The best food sources for this level of deficiency are liver, whole organic eggs, and red meat. Wild game and duck are particularly rich. Also, take dessicated liver capsules (organic buffalo liver is best—if unavail-able call 1-800-243-5242), 6 caps twice daily. This is an easy way to gain natural liver-source niacin. Strictly avoid all alcoholic bev-erages and refined sugars. Alcohol is a primary cause of niacin deficiency. Constant drinking causes catastrophic damage to internal organs, specifically as a result of niacin deficiency.

Vitamin B-5 (Pantothenic Acid)

Pantothenic acid was discovered in 1933 by the noted American biochemist Roger Williams. Dr. Williams found that animals deprived of vitamin B-5 developed a variety of degenerative diseases and eventually died. After many years of research on pantothenic acid, Dr. Williams concluded that the vitamin was commonly deficient in the American diet. In his words, "it is wishful thinking to suppose that people always get enough (from their diets)." Further, Dr. Williams provided convincing data that humans require as much as twice the pantothenic acid as animals. What's more, he clearly documented the heightened need for B-5 in individuals suffering from constant psychological stress. Thus, it is no surprise that soon after he published his research, pantothenic acid became known as the "anti-stress vitamin".

Pantothenic acid should also be nicknamed "the power vitamin". That is because a deficiency of this vitamin results in weakness and/or fatigue, and supplementation with it usually leads to an immediate increase in vitality and strength. It makes sense that pantothenic acid would have this effect. It is required for the synthesis of adrenal hormones, and these hormones are responsible for the human body's ability to cope with the normal stresses of existence and the abnormal ones as well.

The adrenal glands produce dozens of hormones, each of which is an essential component of the stress-coping mechanism. These hormones are also involved in the maintenance of normal body functions, such as salt and water retention, blood sugar regulation, anti-inflammatory activity, calcium and magnesium metabolism, libido, and immune activation.

Stress rapidly depletes tissue stores of pantothenic acid. Without adequate amounts of this vitamin the stress-induced deficiency of adrenal hormones becomes extreme. A severe deficiency of adrenal hormones may lead to a potentially fatal disease, known as Addison's disease. More commonly, individuals suffer from the debilitating but rarely fatal condition called subclinical Addison's disease. This condition results in such a wide range of symptoms that it is often underdiagnosed by physicians. This is unfortunate, since untold millions of Americans suffer from this debilitating condition.

Millions of Americans suffer from extreme and prolonged psychological stress. It is crucial to realize that the invaluable and life-preserving adrenal hormones are "used up" by stress. People who have endured prolonged stress are usually severely deficient in both pantothenic acid and adrenal hormones. What's more, prolonged stress, as might occur from grieving, chronic health problems, and/or marital discord, can damage the adrenal glands, but only if a deficiency of pantothenic acid exists. This illustrates how crucial it is to maintain adequate tissue stores of the vitamin. Regular supplementation with pantothenic acid can help reverse stress-induced adrenal damage.

One particularly amazing feature of pantothenic acid is that a deficiency can cause symptoms to develop rather rapidly. Usually, it takes several months or perhaps years for a deficiency of a nutrient to surface in the form of symptoms and/or ailments. In contrast, vitamin B-5 deficiency may cause symptoms to occur within days. Researchers discovered that a whole catalog of illnesses and symptoms resulted when pantothenic acid was selectively removed from the diet of human volunteers. Perhaps the most dominating finding was the damage that occurs to the adrenal glands. The researchers discovered that this damage was particularly acute if the adrenal glands were already severely stressed. Stress combined with pantothenic acid deficiency resulted in cell death within the glands. As a result, the ability of the glands to produce adrenal hormones was severely impaired. However, when the diet was supplemented with pantothenic acid, the damage was prevented and the function returned to normal.

Unfortunately, pantothenic acid is found in large amounts in relatively few foods. Top sources include organ meats, egg yolks, muscle meats, soybean flour, and royal jelly. Fruits, pasta, vegetables, and most beans are devoid of pantothenic acid. Thus, strict vegetarians frequently develop B-5 deficiencies.

VITAMIN B-5 (PANTOTHENIC ACID) TEST

Which of these apply to you?

1. chronic fatigue
2. fall asleep more easily sitting up
3. insomnia
4. bloating and/or distension after eating
5. rapid pounding of heart/pulse on exertion
6. burning feet and/or heels
7. hard pebble-like stools
8. chronic constipation
9. vague abdominal pains
10. nervousness
11. mood swings
12. anxiety and/or panic attacks
13. depression
14. extreme weakness
15. muscle cramps, especially cramps in the feet or toes
16. quarrelsome or hot-tempered behavior
17. low blood pressure
18. susceptibility to infections, especially sore throats
19. patchy hair loss (alopecia)
20. lack of coordination
21. faintness or fainting spells (blackouts)
22. crying spells
23. nausea and/or vomiting
24. eczema and/or psoriasis
25. jumpiness and/or shakiness
26. noise sensitivity
27. headaches
28. food allergies
29. sensitivity to chemicals

30. infrequent urination
31. compulsive behavior
32. inability to cope with stress
33. excessive sweating of palms and feet
34. impaired memory
35. pains in the lower neck and upper back
36. receding gums
37. vague abdominal pain
38. lack of appetite
39. restless leg syndrome (constant motion of legs at night)
40. bruxism (grinding of the teeth and clenching of the jaw at night)
41. sleep apnea
42. sleepiness during the day
43. agitation and/or temper tantrums
44. Do you take cortisone and/or use cortisone creams?
45. Have you been under severe stress recently?
46. Do you have a history of severe allergic disease such as hives, eczema, and/or asthma?
47. Do you consume alcohol on a regular basis (one or more drinks per day)?
48. Do you have chronic joint pain?
49. Do you have a history of TMJ syndrome?
50. Do you suffer from frequent outbreaks of herpes (cold sores, genital herpes, shingles)?
51. Do you have chronic pain in the mid to lower back that is described as "kidney pain?"
52. Is your hair turning gray prematurely?
53. Do you suffer from diabetes or hypoglycemia?
54. Do you have a history of gout attacks?
55. Do you fall asleep spontaneously or uncontrollably during the day (narcolepsy)?

Your Score _____

---

1 to 9 points *Mild pantothenic acid deficiency*: Take 100 mg of pantothenic acid three times daily. Minimize the consumption of refined sugars and grains. Also, as a potent natural source of B-5 take fortified royal jelly, i.e. Royal Kick, 2 or more capsules daily.

10 to 21 points *Moderate pantothenic acid deficiency*: Take 500 mg three times daily. Increase the consumption of foods rich in pantothenic acid, including royal jelly, bee pollen, organic liver, and fresh meats. Follow a low sugar and starch diet. Reduce the consumption of alcohol and avoid caffeine. Also, as a potent natural source of B-5 take fortified royal jelly, i.e. Royal Kick, 4 or more capsules daily.

22 to 31 points *Severe pantothenic acid deficiency:* Take 1,000 mg three times daily. Avoid refined sugar and severely restrict alcohol intake. Take one teaspoon of royal jelly with breakfast and dinner. Increase the consumption of foods rich in protein and natural fats and reduce your carbohydrate intake. Carbohydrates, particularly refined ones, stress the adrenal glands and increase the demand for pantothenic acid. Curtail the consumption of all dietary sources of refined sugar, white flour, caffeine, and alcohol. As a source of naturally-occuring pantothenic acid take Nutri-Sense, two heaping tablespoons daily. Also, as a potent natural source of B-5 take fortified royal jelly, i.e. Royal Kick, 6 or more capsules daily.

32 and above *Extreme pantothenic acid deficiency*: Warning— extreme debilitation, that is fatigue, weakness, mental derangement, and chronic pain, are likely to develop at this level of deficiency. Prolonged extreme B-5 deficiency may result in the onset of degenerative disease, including arthritis, asthma, immunodeficiency, lupus, heart rhythm disturbances, hypoglycemia, and diabetes. Follow the afore mentioned dietary advice, and take 1,000 mg of pantothenic acid four times daily. If you scored above 42 points, the dosage of pantothenic acid is 2,000 mg 4 times daily (or 2,500 mg three times daily). Ideally, spread out the dosage as much as possible, since this ensures constant stimulation of adrenal steroid synthesis. Additionally, take one teaspoon of royal jelly three times daily; royal jelly is the richest known naturally occurring source of pantothenic acid. Also, as another naturally-occuring source of pantothenic acid, take Nutri-Sense, three heaping tablespoons daily. As a potent natural source of B-5 take fortified royal jelly, i.e. Royal Kick, 6 or more capsules daily. Vitamins A, C, E, and B-6, as well as the minerals selenium, chromium, and magnesium, are extra-important, since they help conserve pantothenic acid. Be sure to take them on a daily basis. Avoid all foods containing refined sugars, and curtail the consumption of alcoholic beverages. Alcohol destroys pantothenic acid. Caffeine weakens the adrenal glands and aggravates the B-5 deficiency state by causing the loss of this nutrient through the urine. All sources of caffeine and caffeine-like substances, such as cocoa, coffee, tea, soft drinks and vanilla bean, should be eliminated from the diet.

Vitamin B-6 (Pyridoxine)

Recent scientific studies indicate that the potential for pyridoxine deficiency in America has been grossly underestimated. As many as 60% of Americans may be severely deficient in the vitamin.

This widespread B-6 deficiency has potentially serious consequences. That is because this vitamin controls a broad range of physiological processes, including enzyme synthesis, fat and carbohydrate metabolism, protein digestion and metabolism, hormone production, and neurotransmitter synthesis. However, its most critical role relates to protein synthesis. The production of virtually all proteins within the human body, of which there are thousands, is dependent upon B-6. Additionally, B-6 is required for the synthesis of the genetic material—DNA and RNA—and, thus, it is an essential nutrient for the reproduction of all cells. What's more, the health of the immune system is dependent upon B-6.

According to Dr. Phillip L. White, former director of the A.M.A's Department of Food and Nutrition, vitamin B-6 "is needed for the production of antibodies as part of the body's immune response." He also notes that it is required for the synthesis of hemoglobin. Both antibodies and hemoglobin are proteins. In addition, research by Axelrod proved that, of all B-vitamins, pyridoxine is the most crucial one for enhancing immune function.

Perhaps of equal importance as its role in protein synthesis is the function of B-6 in fatty acid synthesis. Without B-6, fatty acid metabolism comes to a screeching halt. We can live without protein for weeks or even months (although not without some ill consequences), but a complete deficiency of essential fatty acids, which may occur in association with severe B-6 deficiency, can rapidly lead to life-threatening diseases. (See Essential fatty acid deficiency test, pages 197-203.)

Vitamin B-6 is an invaluable aid in the treatment of a variety of illnesses, including carpal tunnel syndrome, high blood pressure, diabetes, depression, anxiety, and insomnia. Like vitamin C, entire books have been dedicated to elaborating upon the medicinal values of B-6. An example is *The Doctor Who Looked at Hands,* by John Ellis, M.D. He describes the close relation between B-6 deficiency and heart disease. Dr. Ellis provides convincing evidence that the nerves of the heart, as well as the heart muscle itself, become damaged in the event of B-6 deficiency. He also stresses the interrelation between B-6 deficiency and joint disease, describing how the administration of B-6, either by mouth or preferably via injection, rapidly eliminated joint pain and swelling in individuals suffering from arthritis. Further, according to Dr. Ellis the seemingly epidemic problem of fluid retention is due largely to B-6 deficiency. Millions of Americans suffer from this pervasive problem, and women are most vulnerable. Fluid can accumulate in the face, within or under the eyelids, in the fingers and hands, over the sacrum, on the top of the feet, over the abdomen, and in the lower legs. Premenstrual fluid retention is a distressing symptom, and women can gain as much as eight pounds during a single menstrual cycle. Dr. Ellis describes how hundreds of his patients have been relieved of this annoying condition by taking 50 to 100 mg of vitamin B-6 daily.[2]

The digestion and absorption of protein is dependent upon adequate supplies of vitamin B-6. Additionally, this vitamin is required for the formation of a variety of highly specialized nervous system proteins called neurotransmitters. These compounds include adrenaline, noradrenaline, serotonin, GABA, and tryptophan. Other functions of vitamin B-6 include RNA synthesis, hormone synthesis, antibody synthesis, and white blood cell formation.

B-6 is a natural anti-depressant. It is used as an invaluable adjunct in the treatment of chronic mental disturbances. As little as 50 mg per day may produce significant mood elevation. Studies have shown that it can even be helpful in the treatment of notoriously difficult to cure mental disorders, including retardation, anxiety, schizophrenia, mania, sleep disorders, and/or autism. Additionally, B-6 is of value in the treatment of epilepsy, particularly the types that occur in infants and young children. Epilepsy usually responds to megadoses of B-6, and the dosages are often so high that they should be taken only while under a physician's care. The safest form is the coenzyme type, that is pyridoxal-5-phosphate (P5P).

Vitamin B-6 deficiency has been associated with peripheral nerve disorders such as diabetic neuropathy, sciatica, paraesthesia, and carpal tunnel syndrome. Carpal tunnel syndrome may well be the number one complaint in the work-

---

2. Caution: Megadoses of B-6 should be consumed only under a doctor's care. Evidence exists that dosages of B-6 above 100 mg per day may cause temporary and, in some instances, permanent nerve damage.

place today. It's touted as being due solely to the repetitive movement of the hands and arms. While it is largely a mechanical problem, poor diet often initiates the abnormality by inducing B-6 deficiency. However, giving vitamin B-6 alone may not solve this problem. That is because the metabolism of B-6 within nerve fibers is controlled by thyroid hormone. Therefore, defective thyroid function, despite the presence of adequate B-6 levels, can lead to carpal tunnel syndrome. When treated with natural thyroid medication and the appropriate nutrients, especially B-6, there is improvement in the majority of cases, without surgery.

Only a small amount of B-6 is stored in the body, and it is rapidly depleted by stress. Many drugs destroy it, and the list includes aspirin, high blood pressure medicines, cortisone, laxatives, birth control pills, Dilantin, and antibiotics. Additionally, fluorescent light inactivates vitamin B-6. Thus, much of the food in the supermarket is depleted of this vitamin by the time it is consumed. Pyridoxine is water soluble, so much of it is lost when vegetables and other foods are boiled. The following are typical examples of B-6 losses in processed foods:

- white flour: 80%
- white rice: 85%
- canned juice: 40%
- canned vegetables: 60-90%
- preserved meats: 70%
- canned fruits: 50-70%

Of the foods rich in B-6 only poultry and fish are commonly consumed in the American diet. Other excellent food sources include rice bran, brown rice, wheat bran, sunflower seeds, soybeans, and organ meats. Since B-6 foods are rarely eaten in large quantities in the American diet the deficiency is epidemic.

VITAMIN B-6 (PYRIDOXINE) TEST

Which of these apply to you?

1. inability to digest protein
2. indigestion and/or heartburn
3. nausea and/or vomiting
4. acne, particularly whiteheads
5. constipation
6. chronic fatigue and/or exhaustion
7. insomnia
8. mood swings
9. fluid retention
10. nervousness and/or agitation
11. low blood pressure
12. convulsions and/or epilepsy
13. confusion
14. depression
15. seborrheic dermatitis, especially of the face or nose
16. reddened tongue and/or smooth tongue
17. muscular weakness
18. oily hair
19. loss of texture and/or shine of hair
20. premature aging of facial skin
21. irritability
22. bad breath
23. swelling of the face, abdomen, and/or extremities during menses
24. dryness and/or scaling behind the ears
25. poor concentration (or attention deficit disorder in children)
26. dry patches of skin on the face and/or scaly facial skin
27. dry eyes
28. blurred vision
29. excessively dry hair
30. nighttime leg cramps

31. tooth decay
32. tendency to cry easily
33. hair loss
34. lack of dreams or dream recall
35. lips which are constantly chapped
36. enlarged facial pores
37. Are you highly sensitive to MSG?
38. Have you ever been diagnosed with protein in the urine?
39. Do you have an abnormally high cholesterol?
40. Do you have a history of kidney stone formation?
41. Does chronic depression, psychosis, schizophrenia, and/or mania run in the family?
42. Do you regularly take diuretics?
43. Do you regularly consume birth control pills?
44. Do you regularly consume alcoholic beverages (4 or more drinks per week)?
45. Do you regularly take cortisone?
46. Do you currently take antibiotics on a daily, weekly, or monthly basis?
47. Do you have a history of melanoma?
48. Does your skin crack open easily, especially during the winter or as a result of stress?
49. Do you gain weight during or prior to your menstrual period?
50. Do you have a history of carpal tunnel syndrome?
51. Do you have a history of mitral valve prolapse?

Your Score _____

1 to 8 points *Mild B-6 deficiency*: Vitamin B-6 is a nutrient of such vast importance that even a minimal deficiency may produce symptoms. Perhaps the most common result of mild B-6 deficit is a lack of dream recall or no dreams at all. Mental disturbances, such as short-term memory loss and/or depression, may also result. Correct this deficiency by taking a B-complex tablet morning and night and by supplementing the diet with B-6-rich foods.

9 to 19 points *Moderate B-6 deficiency*: At this stage individuals become vulnerable for the development of illnesses due to B-6 deficiency. Such illnesses include depression, anxiety, epilepsy, kidney stones, melanoma, diabetes, PMS, carpal tunnel syndrome, eczema, and heart disease. To correct this deficiency take a B-complex tablet twice daily in addition to 25 mg of B-6 twice daily. Reduce the B-6 dosage by one half after 2 months.

20 to 31 points *Severe B-6 deficiency*: Severe B-6 deficit can result in a variety of symptoms and/or illnesses. Aggressive treatment should include a B-complex tablet taken twice daily along with an additional 50 mg of B-6. Supplement the diet with large helpings of foods rich in B-6, including tuna, salmon, liver, white meat of fowl, nuts, halibut, red meat, and bananas. Reduce the total B-6 dosage to 50 mg once daily after 2 months.

32 and above *Extreme B-6 deficiency*: Extreme B-6 deficit may precipitate a variety of illnesses. B-6 is required for the synthesis of a variety of proteins which are essential to life. Impaired protein synthesis/digestion may contribute to the onset of asthma, migraine headaches, hives, and other allergy-induced diseases. Musculoskeletal conditions, such as fibromyalgia, fibromyositis, back pain, neck pain, carpal tunnel syndrome, and arthritis, also have been correlated with B-6 deficiency and/or impaired protein digestion. Additionally, since B-6 is involved in kidney function, abnormalities involving this system, such as kidney stones, kidney infections, premenstrual edema, peripheral edema, and congestive heart failure, may occur. The brain and nervous system require B-6 for the production of neurotransmitters, for instance, serotonin, acetylcholine, and norepinephrine. Thus, it is no surprise that when tissue levels of B-6 drop to a critical point, depression, anxiety, psychosis, mania, insomnia, and even convulsions (epilepsy) may result. Follow the same recommendations as listed previously, eat plenty of B-6 rich foods (i.e. red meat, chicken, fish, nuts, and the germs of whole grains), and take 100 mg of B-6 three times daily. Reduce this dosage to 100 mg daily after 2 months.[3]

Folic Acid

It is difficult to conceive of a nutrient of greater importance than folic acid. It is involved either directly or indirectly in virtually every chemical reaction occurring within the body.

That is because folic acid controls the very basis of human existence: the growth of cells. All cells depend upon this vitamin for their growth and regeneration. Thus, there is no life without it.

Folic acid deficiency is alarmingly common in the USA, with all age groups being adversely affected. Perhaps of greatest concern are the results of recent scientific studies indicating that as many as 90% of teenagers are consuming less than the RDA of folic acid in their diets. Certain high risk groups, particularly blacks, fare even worse. For instance, an article in the *Journal of the American Dietetic Association* revealed that nearly 100% of black youths in certain schools in Mississippi received less than one-half the RDA for this crucial nutrient. Add to this the fact that many teenagers maintain habits that cause the destruction of folic acid, and it is easy to comprehend why this deficiency is so

---

3. Warning: Studies have shown that dosages of B-6 in excess of 100 mg per day may be associated with nerve damage. Individuals who consume megadoses of B-6 must do so with caution. Be sure to take a B-complex supplement every day if you are taking 50 mg or more of B-6. Take the recommended megadoses (100 mg or more daily) for only as long as it takes to cause symptom improvement, then reduce the dosage to a maintenance level. Dosages above 500 mg per day should be consumed only under a doctor's care. On the positive side B-6 is infinitely safer than aspirin, Motrin, Tylenol, and similar over-the-counter drugs.

widespread and how tissue levels of the vitamin may become dangerously low. Agents which deplete and/or destroy folic acid include alcohol (as little as one drink per day may severely reduce tissue folic acid levels), cigarette smoking, chewing tobacco, stress, antibiotics, aspirin, marijuana, and hard drugs.

The term folic acid was originally derived from the Latin word *folium*, which is also the basis of the English term foliage. Thus, the origin of the word folic acid was due to the fact that this nutrient is commonly found in green edible plants. Actually, it was first isolated from spinach. Research in the 1940s determined that folic acid helped cure two serious diseases: megaloblastic anemia of pregnancy and malabsorptive syndrome (tropical sprue).

Researchers have discovered that folic acid can be utilized as a potent therapy for a variety of degenerative diseases. These diseases include arthritis, cancer (particularly pre-cancerous lesions), alcoholism, anemia, anxiety, depression, pyorrhea, PMS, gout, irritable bowel syndrome, Crohn's disease, ulcerative colitis, heart disease, macular degeneration, cataracts, and atherosclerosis. One notable study was performed to test the ability of folic acid to reverse arterial disease in the elderly. Subjects were given 5.0 to 7.5 mg of folic acid daily. As a result over 90% exhibited improved circulation, plus there was an unexpected benefit: enhanced vision. This was attributed to the localized improvement in circulation within the blood vessels of the eyes. In other words, folic acid helped reverse the aging-induced arterial degeneration which typically occurs within the tiny capillaries that feed the retina. Other studies document how megadoses of folic acid can reverse pre-cancerous lesions of the oral mucosa, lungs, intestines, and uterine cervix.

Top sources of folic acid include organ meats, yeast, chicken, soybeans, rice bran, dark green leafy vegetables, lean beef, veal, eggs, and whole grains. Organically grown foods contain a greater concentration of folates than those grown by commercial farming methods. Pesticides and herbicides destroy folic acid, as do fumigants, which are used to spray fresh produce. Additionally, folic acid is highly sensitive to light, and prolonged storage of food under fluorescent light may lead to a dramatic decline in folate levels. Cooking also destroys this vitamin and as much as 95% may be lost during the preparation of food. The signs are easy to read: Americans are not getting enough folic acid to maintain optimal health, and some individuals are getting so little as to predispose them to a variety of potentially serious diseases.

FOLIC ACID TEST (each response worth 1 point)

Which of these apply to you ?

1. hangnails
2. chronic diarrhea
3. chronic constipation
4. delayed wound healing
5. muscle cramps
6. lack of appetite
7. heartburn and/or indigestion
8. inflammation and/or soreness of the tongue
9. cracks at the corners of the mouth
10. lips which are constantly chapped
11. breathing difficulties
12. insomnia
13. chronic fatigue
14. muscular weakness
15. paranoia
16. depression
17. memory loss
18. growth impairment
19. dry and/or brittle hair
20. slow growing nails and/or hair

21. mouth sores (canker sores)
22. chronic cough (especially smoker's cough)
23. diminished resistance to infection
24. receding and/or bleeding gums
25. chronic gum infections (pyorrhea)
26. Do you eat most of your food canned, cooked, boiled, or fried?
27. Do you have a history of intestinal parasitic and/or fungal infection?
28. Do you have celiac disease and/or wheat allergy?
29. Do you have a history of abnormal pap smears, cervical dysplasia, and/or cervical cancer?
30. Do you have a history of chronic anemia unresponsive to iron or B-12 therapy?
31. Do you have chronic mental illness such as psychosis, anxiety-depression, mania, or schizophrenia?
32. Have you had one or more children with birth defects (spina bifida, etc.)?
33. Do you drink one or more alcoholic beverages daily?
34. Do you smoke cigarettes heavily (one-third pack or more per day), or have you smoked heavily in the past for over five years?
35. Do you use chewing tobacco?
36. Do you smoke cigars or pipes?
37. Do you regularly take birth control pills?
38. Do you take antibiotics on a daily, weekly, or monthly basis?
39. Do you take Dilantin?
40. Do you consume antacids on a daily or weekly basis?
41. Do you take Tagamet or Zantac on a daily or weekly basis?
42. Do you take one or more aspirin daily?
43. Are you on the drug Methotrexate and/or are you under-going chemotherapy?
44. Are you undergoing radiation therapy or have you undergone such therapy recently?

45. Do you have gout?
46. Have you been diagnosed as having reduced protein (globulin, creatinine, or BUN) or low uric acid levels in your blood?

Your Score _____

---

1 to 9 points *Mild folic acid deficiency*: Folic acid is such a crucial nutrient that the functioning of the human body is impaired even in mild deficiency states. To correct the condition, take at least 400 mcg of folic acid daily and increase the consumption of folic acid-rich foods.

10 to 19 points *Moderate folic acid deficiency*: Take a B-complex tablet in addition to 5 mg of folic acid. Eat dark green leafy vegetables on a regular basis. Fresh meats are also an excellent source of folic acid, and to achieve optimal benefits, eat red meat medium rare. Be sure to consume the juices of the meat; this is where most of the folic acid is found. Other excellent sources include brown rice and dark green leafy vegetables. Avoid refined sugar, alcohol, white flour, and caffeine, all of which deplete or destroy folic acid.

20 to 29 points *Severe folic acid deficiency*: Symptoms of folic acid deficiency rapidly dissipate once cellular levels are replenished. To treat this condition aggressively take 10 mg of folic acid daily. Follow the aforementioned dietary advice; in addition, avoid all drugs which destroy folic acid, particularly aspirin. Try the Folic Acid Shake (see the recipe section).

30 and above *Extreme folic acid deficiency*: Warning— damage to internal organs may occur as a result of prolonged, severe folic acid deficiency. Additionally, extreme folic acid deficiency significantly increases the risk for certain types of cancer, notably cervical, colon, and lung cancer. Take 20 mg of folic acid daily. If you scored above 37, take 30 mg daily. Follow the aforementioned dietary advice. Consume absolutely no alcohol. Eliminate refined sugars, white rice, caffeine, and white flour from the diet.

Note: Dosages of 5 mg and above require a prescription from your doctor.

Vitamin B-12

Death and despair were the stimulus for the discovery of vitamin B-12. Until the 1920s pernicious anemia, a relatively common disease of that era, was invariably fatal. Then came the dramatic announcement by Minot and Murphy that large amounts of liver, nearly one pound per day, cured the disease.

Researchers later discovered that liver contains not only large amounts of B-12, but it also stores a unique nutrient called *intrinsic factor*. It was actually this latter substance, which is an essential aid to B-12 absorption, that was responsible for the dramatic improvement of patients with pernicious anemia. By 1955 the most complex of all vitamins was synthesized.

Vitamin B-12 is also known as *cobalamin*. This name was coined after it was discovered that B-12 naturally contains the mineral cobalt. In fact, a cobalt deficiency in the soil may indirectly induce B-12 deficiency within animals.

Dietary vitamin B-12 is found exclusively in foods of animal origin, and the top sources are organ meats, muscle meats, poultry, fish, eggs, and milk products. Seaweed and freshwater algae are the only known plant sources of this vitamin. However, evidence exists that absorption from seaweed and algae is less efficient than animal sources.

B-12 is required for the function of all nerve fibers, particularly the peripheral nerves. Thus, symptoms relative to the function of the brain, spinal cord, nerves, and muscles often dominate the clinical picture of B-12 deficiency.

VITAMIN B-12 TEST (each response worth 1 point)

Which of these apply to you ?

1. dark circles under the eyes
2. chronic fatigue
3. swollen and/or inflamed tongue
4. chronic constipation
5. paranoia and/or psychotic behavior
6. memory loss
7. anemia due to enlarged (macrocytic) red blood cells
8. pale complexion
9. shortness of breath and/or difficulty breathing
10. lack of appetite
11. abdominal discomfort
12. weight loss
13. depression/anxiety
14. burning tongue
15. bursitis
16. bone spurs
17. nervousness, irritability, and/or agitation
18. loss of balance and/or staggering
19. numbness of the hands, legs, or feet
20. confusion
21. loss of taste
22. Have you had your stomach stapled, or has a portion of your stomach been removed?
23. Do you take antacids on a daily or weekly basis?
24. Do you take Tagamet or Zantac on a daily or weekly basis?
25. Do you avoid eating red meats?
26. Are you a vegetarian?
27. Do you regularly consume antibiotics (i.e. six or more dosages per month)?
28. Do you have a history of Crohn's disease, ulcerative colitis, or irritable bowel syndrome?

29. Have you been diagnosed with hypochlorhydria (low stomach acid)?
30. Do you regularly use cortisone or cortisone creams?
31. Have you been diagnosed as having low protein levels in your blood (low globulin, albumin, creatinine, BUN, etc.)?
32. Are you taking birth control pills?
33. Has part of your ileum (lower small intestine) been removed?
34. Do you feel like your feet are too big for your shoes when they really are not?
35. Do you feel like your legs are tight and don't move the way you want them to?
36. Are you over 65 years of age?
37. Do you suffer from premature graying of the hair?

Your Score _____

---

1 to 8 points *Mild vitamin B-12 deficiency*: Take a multiple vitamin-mineral tablet containing B-12 on a daily basis. Increase the consumption of foods rich in B-12, including eggs, liver, lean red meats, and whole milk products. Eat liver at least twice per week. The liver must be derived from organically raised animals free of hormones, pesticides, and other toxic substances. Avoid pork liver.

9 to 18 points *Moderate vitamin B-12 deficiency*: Definitive evidence of B-12 deficiency is difficult to procure even by blood testing. However, blood tests are advisable with this score and should include hemoglobin, red blood cell count, MCH, MCV, MCHC, and a serum B-12 level. The latter test is useful only for individuals who take no B-12 supplements. Follow the previously mentioned advice, but consume the organic liver twice per week for at least one month. Then, eat it once or twice per week. Cook the liver no more than medium or medium rare, otherwise you will inactivate the most biologically active component, i.e. the intrinsic factor. Try also desiccated buffalo liver, six capsules three times daily.

19 to 29 points *Severe vitamin B-12 deficiency*: Warning—if left untreated, prolonged B-12 deficiency may result in permanent damage of the peripheral nerves. B-12 is required for the synthesis of the internal and external components of nerve fibers, including the fatty coating which surrounds the nerves (i.e. the myelin sheath). To correct this condition follow the aforementioned advice. In addition, eat organic liver on a daily basis for at least two months and take eight capsules of desiccated buffalo liver three times daily. No alcohol can be consumed, since it destroys B-12 as well as decreases its absorption. Eliminate refined sugar from the diet. In extreme cases where the absorption of B-12 from foods is compromised, injections may be necessary.

30 and above *Extreme vitamin B-12 deficiency*: Warning— a deficiency producing these symptoms may result in permanent damage to the peripheral as well as spinal nerves. Aggressive medical testing and treatment are probably necessary. See your doctor immediately and request testing for B-12 deficiency. Intramuscular shots of B-12 on a daily or weekly basis are required to rapidly correct this potentially serious condition. In addition, take sublingual or intranasal B-12 (1,000 mcg daily), since these forms are absorbed directly from the tissues into the bloodstream. Also take eight capsules of desiccated buffalo liver four times daily. Oral forms are typically poorly absorbed by individuals with chronic B-12 deficiencies. Folic acid enhances the utilization of B-12. Therefore, folic acid supplementation is also warranted; take at least one milligram of folic acid daily.

Biotin

The essential nature of biotin was discovered by accident. In the 1930s researchers found that animals fed diets containing raw egg whites lost their fur in addition to suffering weight loss, paralysis, and, in some instances, death. The symptoms disappeared when the egg whites were cooked. Later, it was determined that these symptoms were due to biotin deficiency and that the raw egg whites contained a substance which destroyed the naturally occurring biotin in eggs as well as that stored within the tissues.

When biotin deficiency was induced, it created defects in three major areas: the dermatological (hair and skin), neuromuscular (nerves and muscles), and immunological systems. Thus, biotin deficiency can result in significant health impairment. These ill results are because biotin is a crucial component of several human enzyme systems. The biotin-dependent enzymes control such essential functions as protein synthesis, fatty acid synthesis/metabolism, white blood cell activity, and sugar metabolism. The fact that biotin is involved in the synthesis of fatty acids may explain why it is reported to be effective for hair loss, since hair consists largely of protein and essential fatty acids. Biotin is also heavily involved in carbohydrate metabolism.

Recently, researchers discovered that megadoses of biotin are effective in lowering excessively high blood sugar counts, as seen in diabetics. In some diabetics, biotin was so effective in normalizing blood sugar levels that the need for insulin was eliminated.

Like many other B-vitamins, biotin is synthesized by bowel bacteria. Antibiotics, which destroy bowel bacteria, may induce a biotin deficiency state. Good dietary sources of this nutrient include organ meats, egg yolks, legumes, and nuts. Vegetables, fruits, and grains contain little to no biotin.

BIOTIN TEST (each response worth 1 point)

Which of these apply to you?

1. dandruff
2. hair loss (from the scalp)
3. cowlicks (tufts of hair which stand on end)
4. alopecia (patchy hair loss of the scalp)
5. mood swings
6. lack of appetite
7. intolerance to sweets
8. nausea
9. muscle pains/aches
10. weight loss
11. scales on the scalp and/or skin (seborrhea)
12. lassitude
13. depression
14. pallor of the skin and loss of skin pigment
15. delayed development (growth impairment)
16. dry and/or flaky skin
17. brittle hair or hair that breaks easily at the roots
18. lips which are constantly chapped
19. dermatitis (scaly)
20. poor muscle tone and/or muscular atrophy
21. muscular soreness
22. Do you drink alcoholic beverages on a daily or weekly basis?
23. Do you suffer from diabetes or high blood sugar?
24. Do you regularly take antibiotics?
25. Do you eat raw eggs regularly?
26. Do you have abnormally high cholesterol and/or triglyceride levels?
27. Do you consume refined sugar or foods containing sugar on a daily or weekly basis?

28. Do you have hardening of the arteries?
29. Do you have a current and/or family history of male
    pattern baldness?

Your Score ____

---

1 to 7 points *Mild biotin deficiency*: Increase the consumption of biotin-rich foods and take 1 mg of biotin daily. Avoid eating raw eggs.

8 to 15 points *Moderate biotin deficiency*: Take 3 mg of biotin every day. Increase the consumption of biotin-rich foods. Avoid raw eggs as well as refined sugar. Rice polishings and bran are rich in biotin; Take Nutri-Sense, which is a highly digestible type of rice polish/bran, two heaping tablespoons twice daily.

16 and above *Severe biotin deficiency*: At this level of deficiency an individual is vulnerable for the development of diseases/disorders associated with biotin deficit, notably hypoglycemia, diabetes, heart disease, male-pattern baldness, and dermatitis. Take 10 mg of biotin daily. If you are suffering from severe hair loss and/or diabetes, increase the dosage to 10 mg twice daily. Also, take 3 heaping tablespoons of Nutri-Sense, a top source of naturally-occuring biotin, mixed in juice or water, twice daily. Stay on this protocol for at least 90 days, and then reduce the dosage to 5 mg daily. Avoid raw eggs, alcohol, and refined sugar. Add hefty portions of biotin-rich foods to the diet.

Vitamin C

If an individual could choose only one vitamin to take supplementally, it should be vitamin C. Unfortunately, in today's age it isn't easy to get the vitamin C that is required by eating traditional food sources of this nutrient. Even so, many people believe that by eating a helping or two of fresh fruit every day, they are protecting themselves from becoming vitamin C deficient. This is not necessarily true. Furthermore, even though commercial orange juice is thought to be an excellent source of vitamin C, it may contain little or none, that is of the naturally occuring type. That's because cooking, pasteurization, and storage, as well as the addition of synthetic chemicals, destroy much of the vitamin C naturally found in citrus drinks.

Americans live in a world contaminated with a wide range of toxins, and these toxins, whether in the air, water, or food, all destroy vitamin C. What's more, the standard American diet is typically vitamin C deficient, and this is particularly true for those who consume significant amounts of deep fried food, sugar-infested food, and/or junk food. Since the majority of Americans follow such a diet, the fact that over 60% or more of Americans receive less than the RDA for this nutrient should come as no surprise.

Prolonged vitamin C deficiency may result in degenerative changes within a number of tissues, including the joints, spine, spleen, thymus, lymph glands, liver, adrenal glands, ovaries, heart, arteries, veins, testes, and thyroid gland. Vitamin C deficiency may occur within the white blood cells, and this leads to a significant reduction in their microbial killing power. A lack of it also causes a reduction in interferon synthesis, and this chemical is the body's most crucial anti-viral compound.

While scurvy is uncommon today, low-level vitamin C deficit affects millions of Americans. Those at highest risk for such a deficiency include:

- patients taking anticoagulants
- patients who regularly consume cortisone
- patients in chronic pain who consume large amounts of pain killers
- cigarette smokers, their children, and their spouses
- chewing tobacco users
- alcoholics and drug addicts

- nursing home occupants
- individuals on long-term antibiotic therapy
- individuals taking aspirin on a daily or weekly basis

Certain individuals are at a high risk for developing vitamin C deficiency as a result of working around or with noxious compounds. A wide range of compounds destroys or inactivates vitamin C, whether these compounds come in contact with the skin, are ingested internally, or are inhaled (volatile compounds). A list of some of the workers exposed to vitamin C-destroying substances includes:

- tanning salon employees
- gas station attendants
- beauticians
- chemical and nuclear plant employees
- nuclear waste disposal employees
- paper mill workers
- miners
- truck drivers and heavy equipment operators
- oil and gas refinery employees
- employees of synthetic fiber and/or carpet plants
- farmers who work closely with toxic compounds
- dry cleaners
- pressmen
- water/sewage treatment plant employees
- roofers and road asphalt/tar crews
- plastic factory employees
- carpet and/or tile installers
- airline mechanics and ground crews
- flight attendants and airline pilots
- clerks in airports (due to toxic fumes liberated by jets)
- rubber/tire manufacturing plant employees
- battery plant employees
- furniture refinishers

However, despite this extensive problem of toxic chemical exposure, vitamin C deficiency is common in the United States primarily for another reason: the food supply. Less than five percent of the daily caloric intake for Americans comes from fresh uncooked foods. As indicated previously, citrus fruits, unless eaten directly from the tree, are not necessarily vitamin C-rich. Most commercial grapefruits, oranges, and tangerines are picked green and ripened in large warehouses. Incredibly, the ripening agent is bromine gas, which is such a noxious chemical that if it is inhaled in sufficient amounts, it can maim or kill. In contrast, sunlight is a nontoxic ripening agent, which activates or causes the synthesis of vitamin C within the fruit. Thus, because citrus fruits are not tree-ripened, their vitamin C content is reduced significantly. In some instances these fruits contain no measurable amount of this nutrient. What little vitamin C they may originally possess is destroyed by the gas-ripening process as well as by the various fumigants and pesticides that are applied to the fruit prior to shipment. Add to this vitamin losses during transport and storage plus the fact that fluorescent light destroys vitamin C and it can be readily understood that it is possible to purchase citrus fruit devoid of vitamin C.

Gas ripening is so widely practiced by the commercial food and produce industry that only locally grown and/or organic produce can be relied upon as a guaranteed way to receive optimal amounts of dietary vitamin C, that is the amounts listed on food charts. Another option would be to pick your own wild berries and/or fruits or maintain your own fruit trees. However, for the vast majority of Americans that's impractical. Thus, vitamin C supplements must be utilized to fill the void.

To make matters worse Americans are being routinely exposed to a wide range of vitamin C-depleting substances. Anti-vitamin C agents inactivate or destroy the vitamin through a process known as *oxidation*. These oxidative agents include:

- coffee
- sulfites
- nitrates
- cortisone
- antibiotics
- aspirin
- Indocin, Motrin, Voltarin, or Clinoril
- radiation treatments
- antihistamines
- smoke from burning wood
- carbon monoxide
- chemotherapeutic agents
- glue vapors
- X-rays
- refined sugar
- radioactive dyes
- cleansers and degreasers
- black tea
- MSG
- food dyes (synthetic)
- birth control pills
- cigarette, pipe, and cigar smoke
- pesticides
- smoked foods
- chewing tobacco
- natural gas
- inorganic iron
- exhaust fumes
- paint vapors
- microwaves

Negative Vitamin C Balance

As previously indicated millions of Americans receive less than the RDA of vitamin C in their diets. In addition, the dietary habits of Americans, as well as the environments they live in, expose them to a number of substances, which destroy vitamin C. Yet, of all vitamin C antagonists cigarette smoke takes precedence; some 25 million Americans are heavy smokers. Cigarette smoke destroys vitamin C essentially at a more rapid rate than it can be consumed. The smoke from a single cigarette may consume as much as 40 mg of vitamin C. A pack wipes out approximately 700 mg: three packs, 2,000 mg. Virtually no one in this country consumes enough dietary vitamin C to neutralize that many cigarettes. Thus, smokers, even without considering any other vitamin C-destroying factors, suffer from an extremely dangerous condition: totally negative vitamin C status, a condition which leaves them vulnerable to a wide range of severe illnesses, including lung infections, systemic infections, liver disease, blood vessel fragility, heart disease, emphysema, connective tissue breakdown, and, of course, cancer. What's more, most smokers consume large amounts of coffee, refined sugar, and alcohol, all of which oxidize vitamin C.

Passive smokers fair little better. Those who are in the same room with cigarette smokers lose untold millions of molecules of vitamin C every time smokers light up.

Let's look at another example: the business executive who has a high stress job. Stress causes vitamin C to become rapidly consumed within the body and also leads to its loss into the urine. Without vitamin C the body fails to produce enough adrenaline, adrenal steroids, neurotransmitters, and similar substances which maintain normal cellular functions. The preliminary manifestation of this is fatigue. This forces the executive to pursue uppers; he/she uses sugar fixes, coffee, tea, cigarettes, alcohol, and even drugs in an attempt to achieve quick remedies for the tiredness. The morning begins with a cup of black coffee and a sweet roll: a zero vitamin C breakfast. The refined sugar in the sweet roll and the various chemicals in the coffee destroy whatever vitamin C exists in the body. Thus, the executive starts the day with a negative C balance, a nutritionally disastrous circumstance.

To make matters worse the executive arrives at the job only to enter a smoke-filled room. Next, he/she attends a midmorning conference, which happens to be a particularly stressful one. In addition to the cigarette smoke which permeates the air there is a tray of doughnuts, cookies, and plenty of piping-hot coffee. He/she chugs down another cup of coffee and half a doughnut. The vitamin C deficit deepens. Now the executive begins to develop the symptoms of a migraine but thinks it is stress-induced (it is probably due to sugar, coffee, or smoke allergy). Worrying that it might become severe and force him/her to leave work, the executive pops a couple of aspirin. What little vitamin C is left in the tissues is now thoroughly decimated. By noon the pain deepens; perhaps eating will make it feel better, he/she presumes. The executive orders a submarine sandwich with french fries and covers the sub and fries with ketchup. The sub contains salami, a nitrated meat. Nitrates aggressively oxidize vitamin C. Then he/she ingests another dose of aspirin and follows the sub with a cup of coffee. Immediately after lunch, sinus pressure develops; he/she swallows a couple of antihistamines, another drug which destroys vitamin C. To his/her surprise the headache is worse, not better. What's more, the executive is now overwhelmed with severe fatigue and a sort of internal agitation. Migraine pain, fatigue, agitation, and stuffy sinuses all add up to prompt this person to leave work early. This is despite consuming six aspirin, which failed to curb the pain.

Even though the executive is now in the relaxing confines of home, he/she feels overwhelmed because of the stress at work and the stress of the sinus pressure and migraine. The executive was previously informed by a medical professional that alcohol helps digestion. Since his/her stomach is tied in knots, he/she drinks a couple of shots of bourbon before the evening meal. He/she continues to feel miserable, picks at supper, grabs a glass of milk, takes another antihistamine and three more aspirin, then retires for the night: sick, tired, miserable, in pain, stressed, and totally deficient in vitamin C.

Since the migraine will likely continue into the next day or for several additional days, these extreme dietary and drug habits will also be repeated. No one should be surprised if such an individual suddenly drops dead from a heart attack, suffers a stroke, develops a life-threatening bleeding ulcer, or is afflicted with some other severe disease. It should be no surprise if this type of person develops cancer at a young age. Just as vitamin C is destroyed by these dangerous habits, other crucial anti-stress and anti-cancer nutrients, which include vitamin A, beta carotene, vitamin E, B-vitamins, selenium, magnesium and calcium, are also depleted.

The extent of vitamin C deficiency in America can be illustrated by viewing some sample menus. The following pages list typical menus for American adults, teenagers, and children.

Adult's Menu	Vitamin C Content

Breakfast

Bacon and eggs
Commercial cereal sweetened with sugar
Skim milk
Glass of orange juice

total 20 mg

Lunch

Hot dog with bun, ketchup,
  mustard, and sweet relish
French fries
Fudgesicle

total 0 mg

Snack

Can of pop (caffeinated)
Bag of potato chips

total 0 mg

Dinner

Steak cooked well done
Instant mashed potatoes
White bread with butter
Salad made from iceberg lettuce and
  tomato wedges with French dressing
Apple pie al à mode
Cup of coffee with sugar added

total 7 mg

This is an example of a typical middle-class American family menu. The individuals of this "family" only received 27 mg of vitamin C, and this daily ration is less than the RDA. However, as with most American families, the diet contains significant amounts of refined sugars, food additives, caffeinated beverages, junk foods, and refined flours. All of these substances oxidize vitamin C. Individuals who follow this type of diet will develop a negative vitamin C balance, unless their diets are supplemented with several hundred milligrams of vitamin C each day and/or they consume large helpings of fresh, organically-raised fruits with every meal. In this example there are no fresh fruits or vegetables in the menu. The final score is as follows:

a) Coffee: steals 5 mg
b) Sugar (20 tsp per day): steals 20 mg
c) Miscellaneous food additives: steal 10 mg
d) Inorganic iron (in flour products): steals 20 mg
e) Exhaust fumes (from driving to and from work): steal 20 mg

Total Negatives:	-75 mg
Total Positives:	27 mg
Grand Total:	-48 mg

The following is a menu typical for today's teenager:

Teenager's Menu   **Vitamin C Content**

Breakfast

None
(or)
Can of pop and leftover piece of pizza
(or)
Bowl of sugar-sweetened cereal
  with skim milk

                                        total 0 mg

Snack

Ho-Ho, Twinkie, or Suzi-Q

total 0 mg

Lunch

Hamburger with fries (ketchup and onions)
Chocolate malt

total 0 mg

Snack

Apple

total 15 mg

Dinner

Roast beef (well done)
Baked potato with margarine
Canned corn
Orange juice drink (artificial flavors
  and colors; no real juice added)

total 25 mg

This teenager smokes (one-half pack per day), resulting in a loss of 450 mg of vitamin C. His/her diet is high in sugar, and this causes the oxidation of 50 mg. The white flour, with its inorganic iron content, causes a loss of 20 mg. Add to this the typical loss from environmental toxins and exhaust fumes and the total negatives are:

Total Negatives:	-540 mg
Total Positives:	+40 mg
Grand Total:	-500 mg

Now let's look at a typical menu for American children:

Child's Menu	Vitamin C Content

Breakfast

Cereal containing sugar
 (ascorbic acid added)
Skim milk
Glass of apple juice

total 7 mg

Snack

Cookie
Glass of milk

total 0 mg

Lunch

Sloppy Joe with dill pickle slices
French fries
Kool-aid
Small orange

total 12 mg

Snack

Candy bar
Can of pop

total 0 mg

Dinner

Spaghetti-O's
Canned corn
Piece of baked chicken
Chocolate cake
Glass of milk

total 0 mg

Incredibly, the total vitamin C intake for the child in this example is a pitiful 19 mg, which is barely one third of the RDA. To make matters worse this child is consuming a number of substances which oxidize vitamin C, including sugar, inorganic iron, bleached flour, food dyes, artificial flavors, caffeine, MSG, and toxic oils (in the French fries). All told, these noxious agents destroy approximately 60 mg of vitamin C, fully wiping out the daily intake. In addition, the child's parents smoke freely both in the home and car. Add another negative 50 mg, and the negative vitamin C balance for this day becomes - 91 mg.

Total Negatives:	-110 mg
Total Positives:	+ 19 mg
Grand Total:	- 91 mg

In contrast, here is an example of a menu rich in vitamin C:

Menu	Vitamin C Content

Breakfast

2 poached eggs, lightly cooked
Bowl of oatmeal (not overdone) with
 raisins or black currants
Milk or cream
1/2 grapefruit
Mineral water

total 65 mg

Lunch

Fresh vegetable sticks
 (carrots, red peppers, zucchini and/or celery)

All-natural cheese dip
(with non-irradiated spices added)
Poached salmon topped with lemon-butter
 sauce, capers, and pink peppercorns
Rose hip herbal tea

total 130 mg

Snack

Nectarine and glass of mineral water

total 10 mg

Dinner

Salad made of fresh dark greens, including
 romaine lettuce, spinach, green onions,
 and watercress (extra virgin olive oil and
 lemon juice dressing)
Roast beef done medium rare
Baked potato with butter
Steamed broccoli
Bowl of fresh fruits
 (strawberries, kiwi fruit, and blueberries)

total 180 mg

The only negative factor affecting vitamin C status in this example is the unavoidable inhalation of pollutants and exhaust fumes that occurs in a typical day.

Total Negatives:	-20 mg
Total Positives:	+385 mg
Grand Total:	+365 mg

Vitamin C is found in a wide range of foods but is readily destroyed by cooking. Top food sources include rose hips, citrus fruits, spices, bell peppers, broccoli, strawberries, guavas, Brussels sprouts, and dark green leafy vegetables.

VITAMIN C TEST (each response worth 1 point)

Which of these apply to you?

1. easy bruising
2. bleeding and/or purple-appearing gums
3. lower back pain
4. arthritis or other joint pain
5. delayed wound healing
6. loose teeth
7. chronic fatigue
8. sensitivity to extremes in temperature
9. thinning of the bones
10. nosebleeds
11. thinning and/or premature aging of the skin
12. liver spots
13. petechiae (tiny red blood spots in the skin)
14. heightened susceptibility to infections
15. hemorrhoids
16. insomnia
17. dryness of the mouth
18. dry, itching skin
19. swollen joints
20. loss of appetite
21. listlessness and/or apathy
22. depression
23. tendency to form plaque and/or tartar
24. Do you regularly consume aspirin?
25. Do you regularly take non-steroidal anti-inflammatory agents such as Motrin, Indocin, Clinoril, or Butazolidin?
26. Do you regularly consume birth control pills?
27. Do you take antibiotics on a daily or weekly basis?
28. Are you exposed to excessive quantities of chemical or exhaust fumes while on the job or during your travels?
29. Do you eat a limited quantity of fruits and vegetables?

30. Do you currently use cocaine, crack, or heroin, or have you used such drugs for prolonged periods in the past?
31. Do you currently consume marijuana, or have you consumed it for prolonged periods in the past?
32. Are you a cigarette smoker?
33. Are you exposed to passive (second-hand) smoke on a regular basis?
34. Do you easily injure your joints, muscles, or tendons?
35. Do you take cortisone or apply cortisone cream on a daily or weekly basis?
36. Do you suffer from learning or reading impairment?
37. Do you have a history of hardening of the arteries?
38. Do you work in or near a nuclear facility/power plant, or are you exposed on a monthly basis to x-rays?
39. Do you see spots ("floaters") in your eyes?
40. Do you have a history of degenerative joint disease?
41. Do you suffer from growing pains (children/adolescents)?
42. Do you have deep pain in the bones and/or joints?

_____

Your Score ____

_____

1 to 7 points *Mild vitamin C deficiency*: The symptoms of vitamin C deficiency are often vague. However, to be on the safe side take 500 mg of vitamin C twice daily and increase the consumption of foods rich in vitamin C. Also, take a natural vitamin C supplement, such as Flavin-C, 2 capsules daily.

8 to 16 points *Moderate vitamin C deficiency*: Even with a moderate deficiency of vitamin C, collagen production is adversely affected. This leads to skin aging and cellulite production. Take a natural vitamin C supplement, such as Flavin-C, 4 capsules twice daily. Take also 500mg of regular vitamin C. Increase the intake of foods rich in vitamin C. Avoid refined sugar and reduce the intake of caffeine and alcohol. If you are a smoker, it is critical that you quit now in order to prevent further tissue damage.

17 to 26 points *Severe vitamin C deficiency*: At this level of deficiency a wide range of degenerative diseases may occur. These diseases include cancer, heart disease, arthritis, lupus, diabetes, and lung disease. Smokers must understand that if they don't stop their destructive habits now, they may ultimately develop cancer or heart disease. Or, they may be stricken with a severe debilitating lung disease such as emphysema. Follow the previously mentioned dietary advice and take 1,000 mg of vitamin C twice daily. Plus, take large amounts of natural vitamin C, such as Flavin-C, 4 or more capsules twice daily.

27 and above *Extreme vitamin C deficiency*: Warning—damage to critical internal organs is imminent unless the vitamin C deficiency is corrected. Take 1,000 mg of vitamin C twice daily. The frequent dosage is necessary to maintain consistently high blood levels. If the symptoms of vitamin C deficiency persist, greatly increase the intake of natural vitamin C, for instance, drink a quart of freshly squeezed orange or grapefruit juice daily. Also, take Flavin-C, 4 capsules three times daily. Consume large helpings of foods rich in vitamin C and strictly avoid all substances which destroy it.

Vitamin A

Vitamin A is perhaps the most versatile and valuable of all nutrients. An entire book could be written about it, as it serves seemingly innumerable functions within human tissues.

Dietary vitamin A comes from both plant and animal sources. The type found in animals is vitamin A, while plants contain beta carotene, which is essentially two vitamin A molecules bound together by a chemical bond.

Animals cannot make vitamin A. They get it from eating plants. The beta carotene from plants, once absorbed, is split apart by enzymes within animal intestines to form vitamin A.

As many as 60% of Americans suffer from vitamin A deficiency, and if the deficiency becomes extreme, frank symptoms may occur. The widespread consumption of deep fried foods and various refined vegetable oils in the typical American diet is a major reason that the deficiency is so common. Refined oils destroy vitamin A both in the body and within the foods in which they are contained (see the Hydrogenated Oil and Deep Fried Oil test).

To optimally utilize dietary vitamin A it is necessary to have an adequately functioning liver. The liver performs several crucial functions in respect to the digestion, absorption, and distribution of vitamin A, which are listed as follows:

a)   It is the storage depot for both vitamin A and beta carotene. Over 90% of the body's vitamin A is found in the liver.

b)   It is responsible for splitting stored beta carotene into vitamin A upon demand by the tissues.

c)   It stimulates the production of bile, which is needed to unleash vitamin A, as well as other fat-soluble vitamins, from fatty foods.

d)   It synthesizes the carrier protein, retinol binding globulin, without which the absorption of vitamin A becomes virtually impossible.

Vitamin A is essential for the maintenance of optimal immunity. Immune cells, as well as organs such as the thymus and spleen, degenerate in the event of vitamin A deficiency. The adrenal and thyroid glands are also highly sensitive to a decline in vitamin A levels; cellular death within these organs may occur if the deficiency becomes extreme.

Children are particularly vulnerable for developing immune disorders due to a lack of vitamin A, since their diets are often devoid of foods rich in vitamin A. Dr. Lendon Smith, a noted pediatrician and author, relates that children who seem to "catch everything that goes around" usually have significant vitamin A deficiencies.

Since vitamin A is found in two separate forms, it is widely distributed in foods. Top dietary sources include fish liver oils, liver, halibut, salmon, swordfish, crab, butter, cream, whole milk, whole milk cheeses, egg yolks, sweet potatoes, apricots, tomatoes, carrots, dark green leafy vegetables, peaches, dark cherries, red bell peppers, red hot peppers, cantaloupe, winter squash, and pumpkin.

VITAMIN A TEST (each response worth 1 point)

Which of these apply to you?

1. weak or brittle nails
2. brittle hair
3. dry scaly skin
4. goose-bump like lesions on the back of the upper arms
5. acne, especially of the upper back and/or shoulders
6. lack of sense of smell
7. dry hair
8. increased susceptibility to infections
9. night blindness
10. growth impairment and/or short stature
11. thick, scaly patches of the skin and/or mucous membranes
12. poor coordination and/or loss of equilibrium
13. xerophthalmia (dry cornea syndrome; dry eyes)
14. dry mouth
15. slow growing hair and/or nails
16. inflammation of the eyes and/or sties
17. loss of taste
18. weight loss

19. loss of appetite
20. chronic diarrhea
21. conjunctivitis (inflammation and/or redness of the whites of the eyes)
22. Do you have poor fat assimilation/digestion, and/or do you avoid fatty foods?
23. Are you vulnerable to developing infections such as sore throats, ear aches, colds, or flu?
24. Do you consume one or more alcoholic beverages per day?
25. Are you exposed to excessive amounts of sunlight?
26. Do you consume deep fried foods on a daily or weekly basis?
27. Do you have or frequently develop open wounds that become infected such as varicose ulcers, diabetic ulcers, or bed sores?
28. Do you have a history of infertility?
29. Do you use mineral oil as a laxative on a regular basis?
30. Are you currently taking cholesterol-lowering medications?
31. Are you taking prescription drugs which inactivate vitamin A, e.g. Coumadin, Synthroid, Motrin, Indocin, Voltarin, and phenobarbital?
32. Are you taking iron pills or multiple vitamins containing iron on a daily basis?
33. Do you take aspirin on a daily or weekly basis?
34. Do you have a history of nasal polyps?
35. Do you have diabetes?
36. Do you have a history of malabsorptive syndrome, colitis, or Crohn's disease?
37. Do you have a history of chronic pancreatic or liver disease?
38. Do you frequently develop corns and/or calluses?
39. Do you have a history of internal and/or skin cancer?
40. Do you have a history of diabetes?
41. Do you have hypothyroidism?
42. Are you currently taking birth control pills or have you taken them for five or more years in the past?
43. Are you unable to produce tears?

44. Do you have ulceration of the cornea?
45. Are your gums inflamed and/or sore?

Your Score _____

---

1 to 9 points *Mild vitamin A deficiency*: Vitamin A deficiency at any level must be regarded seriously. Treatment includes taking a multiple-vitamin tablet containing vitamin A (10,000 I.U.) plus an additional 10,000 IU. of beta carotene. Be sure to increase the consumption of vitamin A-rich foods.

10 to 19 points *Moderate vitamin A deficiency*: In addition to increasing the consumption of vitamin A-rich foods, take 20,000 I.U. of vitamin A and 25,000 I.U. of beta carotene daily. Avoid refined sugar and alcohol. Eliminate refined vegetable oils and/or margarine. Butter is superior, because it contains this vitamin. Extra virgin olive oil and/or unrefined rice bran oil are acceptable alternatives. Be sure to get your daily fix (or several fixes) of vitamin A and/or beta carotene-rich foods.

20 and above *Severe vitamin A deficiency*: A variety of serious ailments are associated with prolonged vitamin A deficit. These illnesses include immune deficiency, growth retardation, osteoporosis, heart disease, atherosclerosis, emphysema, kidney disease, diabetes, prostate disorders, and arthritis. In addition, numerous eye diseases may be induced as a result of poor vitamin A nurture. These diseases include corneal ulcers, conjunctivitis, night blindness, myopia, ulcerations, macular degeneration, and even blindness itself. In fact, long-standing vitamin A deficiency is the number one cause of blindness in the world. To correct severe vitamin A deficiency, consume liver, the richest known source of vitamin A. Only organically-raised animals should be used as a source of liver. Lamb's liver is the richest edible source and is usually less contaminated than beef or calves' liver. The liver should be cooked as gently as possible to avoid destruction of the vitamin A molecules. Eat it as often as you can, preferably every day for at least a month. In addition, take a multiple vitamin tablet containing at least 20,000 I. U. of vitamin A plus 50,000 I. U. of beta carotene daily. If you cannot eat liver or have no access to organically-raised liver, take 30,000 I. U. of vitamin A, preferably from fish liver oils, each day for two months, then reduce the dosage to a maximum of 20,000 I.U. daily. Do not take large doses of vitamin A for prolonged periods. It is one of the few nutrients which can cause cumulative toxicity.[4]

Vitamin D

The term "vitamin D" is a misnomer. That is because vitamin D is in reality a hormone, not a vitamin. The definition of a vitamin is "an essential nutrient that must be obtained from the diet." This definition fails to apply to "vitamin" D, since it can be synthesized in the human body, specifically in the skin. Known as the "sunshine vitamin", the D hormone, as it should be renamed, is synthesized as a consequence of the interaction of ultraviolet light with skin cells. When the light rays strike the skin, they provoke the synthesis of vitamin D from cholesterol, the latter being located in large quantities within the skin's oil

---

4.   Warning: Vitamin A supplements, including cod liver oil, must not be taken by women of childbearing age. The consumption of vitamin A supplements in megadose quantities during the first trimester of pregnancy has been associated with a variety of birth defects. If you are a woman with child bearing potential, only the standard quantity of vitamin A, as found in multiple vitamins (10,000 IU. daily), can be deemed safe. However, that vitamin A supplements are safe to consume after pregnancy is well established, that is 100 days after conception. A safer approach for women of childbearing years would be to consume natural sources of vitamin A such as organic liver and fatty fish (from unpolluted waters).

glands. Once synthesized, the vitamin is absorbed into the blood or may remain within the skin. As little as one-half hour of sunshine per day may fulfill an individual's vitamin D needs. In contrast, deep dark tans may actually diminish vitamin D production, since excess sun exposure damages the skin cells which produce this nutrient.

Ideally, vitamin D should be included in the diet, even if the individual gets an adequate amount of sunlight. Top dietary sources include milk, egg yolks, cheese, sardines, mackerel, herring, salmon, tuna, halibut, and fish liver oils.

Unfortunately, over the last 30 years seemingly as much emphasis has been placed upon the potential toxicity of vitamin D as its benefits. As a result, the medical profession has neglected to emphasize the crucial role played by this substance in human nutrition. Only in the past decade have physicians and researchers begun to give it the credit it deserves. Recent research has revealed that vitamin D is of value in the treatment of psoriasis, eczema, osteoporosis, arthritis, hypertension, kidney disease, prostate disorders, and heart disease. While synthetic forms, such as those found in many food supplements and the type currently added to milk, may be toxic in high dosages, the natural forms are essentially nontoxic. One major reason for this is the fact that it is virtually impossible to achieve toxic dosages of vitamin D from eating food. There is an exception to this rule: cod liver oil. While the vitamin D in it is natural, one can overdose on it. However, the epidemic problem is vitamin D deficiency, not excess. In fact, recent research indicates that there is more reason to be concerned about the synthetic vitamin D added to milk products than the extra amounts individuals might be getting from cod liver oil or other natural vitamin D supplements. Even so, a teaspoonful of cod liver oil per day is a sufficient dosage for most adults.

There is another type of vitamin D of which to be wary: ergocalciferol. This synthetic version has the greatest toxicity of all types of vitamin D. It is produced in chemistry labs via the irradiation of cholesterol. Do not use supplements containing it. Look for cholecalciferol instead. The latter type is essentially the same as the one produced within the skin.

All of the vitamin D synthesized in the body is made from cholesterol. Therefore, diets low in cholesterol may cause and/or contribute to vitamin D deficiency. This brings into question the value of low cholesterol diets. Cholesterol is an essential nutrient without which a variety of normal physiological functions become impaired. In fact, vitamin D is one of numerous essential compounds produced from cholesterol. These compounds include estrogen, progesterone, testosterone, aldosterone, vitamin K, and cortisone. In the case of a cholesterol restricted diet, deficiencies of all of these life-giving substances are bound to occur. Individuals placed on reduced cholesterol diets who are also taking cholesterol-lowering medications, such as Questran, Pravachol, or Lovistatin, are at the greatest risk for the development of cholesterol deficiency and, therefore, vitamin D deficiency. Tens of millions of Americans currently adhere to low cholesterol diets, and many of these individuals concurrently take cholesterol-lowering medications. All are at a high risk for diseases due to cholesterol deficiency, including cancer, diabetes, dementia, osteoporosis, lupus, adrenal insufficiency, immune deficiency, prostatitis, and even heart disease itself. One of the greatest ironies in modern nutrition is the fact that recent evidence indicates that a fanatical restriction of dietary cholesterol may actually increase the risk of heart disease, particularly in women. This is thought to be due to a severe reduction in the production of certain cholesterol dependent hormones, especially vitamin D, progesterone, and estrogen. Additionally, vegetarians and macrobiotic adherents frequently develop cholesterol and vitamin D deficiencies, since their diets usually omit or restrict meats, fish, milk products, and eggs, the primary natural sources of these nutrients. There are no vegetable sources of vitamin D.

Vitamin D is the missing link in the prevention of osteo-porosis. It also helps prevent arthritis and may be useful in the treatment of this dreaded condition. Its role in these and other bone diseases is based upon the fact that vitamin D is the key nutrient for stimulating the absorption and metabo-lism of calcium. However, there is much more at stake as a consequence of vitamin D's control over calcium metabolism than maintaining strong bones. After all, it is calcium which stimulates the firing of the nerves. It is calcium which mod-ulates the contraction of muscles, notably the heart muscle. It is calcium which maintains strong teeth. It is calcium which helps keep the blood clotting mechanism in balance so that blood is neither too thick nor thin. It is calcium which helps control the growth of the cells.

In respect to its role in cellular growth there is mounting evi-dence that vitamin D helps prevent colon cancer. Researchers at the University of California discovered that people who con-sume vitamin D in their diets, in this instance by drinking milk, were 30% less likely to develop colon cancer compared to peo-ple with similar diets who drank no milk. The researchers emphasized the vitamin D content of milk as the likely reason for this lowered cancer risk.

Vitamin D's role in vision was recently discovered by New York ophthalmologist Arthur A. Knapp. He gave a group of patients the nutrient for several months. The result was that nearsightedness declined in over a third of his patients, and in many patients it was completely corrected. Dr. Knapp's conclusions were that deficiencies of both vitamin D and cal-cium potentiated visual decline as well as the formation of cataracts.

Vitamin D deficiency is common in the United States, and in certain high risk groups it is virtually guaranteed. These groups include invalids, mentally deranged individuals and/or inmates of mental institutions, nursing home patients, pregnant women, strict vegetarians, individuals with chronic kidney disease and/or dialysis patients, people living amidst heavy smog, and individuals who have been bedridden for prolonged periods. All these groups have in common reduced vitamin D synthesis from a lack of exposure to sunlight and/or lowered dietary intake. Other high risk groups include allergic individuals who avoid eggs or milk products (milk products are a prime source of vitamin D) and individuals who rarely consume fatty fish. Additionally, the absorption and metabolism of vitamin D declines dramatically with age. Thus, it is usually advisable that individuals over 50 years of age take a daily dose of supplemental vitamin D, preferably from fish liver oil[5], this especially being true for those who fail to get adequate sunlight. As little as one-half hour of sunlight daily may be sufficient to generate the minimum requirement for vitamin D. The best food sources of vitamin D include yogurt, cheese, butter, liver, and fatty fish.

---

5. **Warning:** Be wary of consuming cod liver oil that has an excessively fishy odor; it may be rancid. If fresh, the smell will not be overpowering. Be sure to refrigerate the oil after opening. To prevent rancidity add 400 I.U. of vitamin E to the bottle, or a few drops of wild oregano (Oreganol).

VITAMIN D TEST

Which of these apply to you (each response worth 1 point)?

1. insomnia
2. irritability
3. rapid heartbeat and/or irregular heartbeat
4. nearsightedness
5. nosebleeds
6. chronic diarrhea
7. bone pain, especially in the legs
8. chronic upper or lower back pain
9. aching in the teeth
10. frequent fractures
11. cataracts
12. premature graying of the hair
13. scoliosis
14. muscular rigidity
15. muscle twitching
16. muscle cramps and/or spasms
17. convulsions and/or seizures
18. vague or migrating joint pain
19. easy bruising
20. soft teeth and/or tooth decay
21. thinning of the bones (osteoporosis)
22. chipping and/or cracking teeth
23. arthritis
24. delayed wound healing
25. bruxism (grinding of the teeth)
26. Do you have psoriasis and/or eczema?
27. Are you bedridden, or were you bedridden for prolonged periods in the past?
28. Do you have fair skin?
29. Do you avoid eating fatty fish such as salmon, halibut, mackerel, sardines, and herring?
30. Are you a vegetarian? (if vegan, add 3 additional points)

31. Do you avoid milk products because of allergy or other reasons?
32. Do you have mitral valve prolapse and/or heart arrhythmia?
33. Do you have colon or prostate cancer?
34. Do you have high blood pressure?
35. Do you have acne, pityriasis, and/or rosacea?
36. Do you get little or no exposure to sunlight?
37. Do you have liver or pancreatic disease?
38. Do you take Dilantin or phenobarbital (epilepsy drugs) on a daily basis?
39. Do you live in an area where there is heavy air pollution?
40. Are you bowlegged?
41. Do you have an excessively high or low serum calcium level?
42. Do you have a low serum phosphorous level?
43. Do you adhere to a low-fat low-cholesterol diet?
44. Do you have a history of duodenal ulcer, or has your duodenum been removed?
45. Do you take Tagamet, Zantac and/or antacids on a regular basis?
46. Do you have celiac disease or gluten intolerance?
47. Do you suffer from muscular weakness?
48. Do you have difficulty walking or climbing stairs?
49. Do you have congestive heart failure or enlarged heart?
50. Do you have gallstones, and/or have you had your gall-bladder removed?
51. Do you have chronic kidney disease?
52. Do you have a cholesterol level below 155 mg/dl?
53. Have you been diagnosed with Osgood-Schlatter disease?
54. Do you have bone cancer?
55. Do you have a concave (pigeon) breast?

Your Score _____

---

1 to 9 points *Mild vitamin D deficiency*: Eat foods rich in vitamin D on a daily basis and take a multiple vitamin containing vitamin D. Be sure to get sun exposure daily.

10 to 21 points *Moderate vitamin D deficiency*: Follow the previously mentioned advice and take an additional 400 I.U. of vitamin D daily. Eat a can of sardines or herring every day. Take a teaspoon of cod liver oil daily. Be sure to get regular sunlight exposure; at least one-half hour per day and no more than 4 hours per day would be ideal. Wear appropriate protective clothing; do not sunbathe for prolonged periods.

22 to 34 points *Severe vitamin D deficiency*: Consume hefty helpings of foods rich in vitamin D (fortified milk products, fatty fish, and eggs) and take 800 I.U. of vitamin D each day. Or, take a tablespoon of cod liver oil daily for one or two months, reducing this dosage to a teaspoonful daily afterwards. Eating fish rich in vitamin D is preferable to consuming cod liver oil, as the oil may become rancid with time. Be sure to get one-half hour or more of sunlight each day, or preferably, one half hour twice daily.

35 and above *Extreme vitamin D deficiency*: Warning—you are at risk for osteoporosis and may suffer spontaneous bone fractures. Softening of the skeleton already may be evident. Furthermore, a long-term vitamin D deficiency greatly increases the risk of cardiac disease, neuromuscular disorders, colon cancer, and bone cancer. Since fat malabsorption is the most common cause of extreme vitamin D deficiency, take the following supplements to improve fat absorption: Lipase 4 capsules (500 mg) with each meal; biotin 5-10 mg three times daily; inositol 1 gm three times daily; granular lecithin 1 heaping tablespoon with meals. Eat foods rich in vitamin D on a daily basis. In addition, take 2,000 I.U. of vitamin D daily for at least two months, reducing the dosage to 1,000 I.U. as a maintenance dosage. Try to get a minimum of one hour of sunlight daily, or preferably, one half hour twice daily.

Vitamin E

Perhaps best known as the fertility vitamin, this nutrient is far more valuable than simply acting as a virilizing agent. Vitamin E is one of the body's most crucial antioxidants, acting to neutralize a variety of toxins before they can cause cellular damage. It is an invaluable aid for the prevention of a variety of diseases. In fact, research has determined that it may prove beneficial for even the chronic so-called incurable diseases such as arthritis, lupus, heart disease, Parkinson's disease, multiple sclerosis, and cancer.

Vitamin E is the key antioxidant for protecting cellular membranes. It readily dissolves into the fatty layer of cell membranes and, once there, acts to protect the membranes from potentially damaging compounds. This function illustrates the tremendous value of vitamin E in living organisms, since, once cell membranes are damaged, the cells usually die or become functionally incompetent.

The NASA astronaut fatigue syndrome is an excellent example of the cellular damage that can occur due to vitamin E deficiency. While in outer space, the astronauts are exposed to dangerously high amounts of radiation from the sun. They have no earthly atmosphere to protect them from the sun's potent ultraviolet rays. These rays pierce the astronauts' tissues like so many billions of microscopic sabers. Inevitably, the astronauts' cells absorb large amounts of this ultraviolet radiation, and tissue damage occurs. The result is sick, tired astronauts.

The fatigue the astronauts experienced is somewhat like that seen in anemic patients. Researchers at NASA discovered that the astronauts were indeed anemic, and the cause was red blood cell membrane destruction by ultraviolet light. When the astronauts' diets were supplemented with vitamin E, this harmful reaction was halted, and the astronaut sickness syndrome disappeared.

Every year vitamin E is the subject of thousands of research articles. There seems to be no limit to the utility of this substance in the treatment and prevention of disease. Research has determined that this vitamin exerts the following functions:

- It protects the digestive tract against cancer-causing chemicals.
- It reverses the damage induced by toxic chemicals, such as carbon monoxide, sulfur dioxide, and petro-chemical fumes, on the lungs and other tissues.
- It protects the skin from sunlight-induced damage.
- It helps prevent eye damage from aging, excessive sunlight, and toxic chemical exposure. Individuals who regularly take supplemental vitamin E are significantly less likely to develop cataracts than those who take no supplements.
- It prevents arterial and heart tissue damage due to aging or toxic chemical ingestion.
- It halts breast tissue damage from the ingestion of toxic fats (polyunsaturated fats; deep-fried oils) and helps reverse fibrocystic breast disease.
- It blocks the growth of certain tumors (in the test tube), notably melanoma.
- It increases blood flow to the internal organs, prevents sludging of the blood, and enhances the heart's pumping ability.
- It increases virility by boosting sperm count and enhancing the fertilization process.
- It prevents cellular membrane damage from dietary toxins such as alcohol, cigarette smoke, and polyunsaturated fats.
- It helps prevent bleeding disorders, such as placental hemorrhaging, menorrhagia (heavy menses), and nose bleeds, by normalizing blood clotting.

Vitamin E is chemically classified as a terpene. Terpenes are alcohol-like substances which readily dissolve in fat. That is why vitamin E is known as a fat-soluble antioxidant, and this is also why it is found primarily in fatty foods. A secondary source is dark green leafy vegetables. Top food sources include almonds, sunflower seeds, hazelnuts, avocados, cold-pressed nut/seed oils, salmon, and spinach.

Since vitamin E is found in significant amounts in relatively few foods, supplements are a convenient means of achieving optimal dosages. People living in industrialized countries need to take a minimum of 400 I.U. daily just to protect themselves from the ill effects of pollution. Individuals who are exposed to noxious chemicals in the work environment or heightened levels of toxins as a result of urban living should take larger doses: 800 to 1600 I.U. daily. One study determined that 800 I.U. was barely enough to neutralize the toxic effects of environmental pollutants and dietary polyunsaturates, which deplete tissue stores of vitamin E. Natural vitamin E is the finest supplemental source, and even though synthetic vitamin E offers the advantage of being less expensive, it is far less effective.[6]

Yet another issue is the extraction of Vitamin E from genetically engineered soy. This type of vitamin E may cause allergic toxicity. Although lower in dosage, stabilized raw pumpkinseed oil, that is Pumpkinol, can be taken as an alternative. 2 to 3 tablespoons daily. This provides about 20 I.U. of crude all-natural vitamin E, the entire complex.

Children are being exposed to higher levels of radiation than ever before in history. Most significant is medical exposure, for instance, asthmatics who undergo repeated chest x-rays. Of even greater consequence is a history of being x-rayed while still in the womb. Millions of women are x-rayed while they are knowingly pregnant or during the early stages of pregnancy before they are aware of the pregnancy. Other sources of childhood radiation exposure include:

---

6. Acceptable forms of natural source vitamin E include mixed tocopherol concentrate, alpha tocopherol, d-alpha tocopherol, vitamin E succinate, and vitamin E acetate. Other high quality sources include food concentrates such as crude pumpkinseed oil (i.e. Pumpkinol). Regarding the letter it is the ideal way to consume natural vitamin E. For further information regarding the definition of quality vitamin E, refer to *How to Eat Right and Live Longer*.

• television and video games
• personal computers
• radioactive dials from toys and/or watches containing radium dyes
• medical x-rays
• radon contamination

Children's diets are notoriously low in vitamin E. White flour, white sugar, white rice, macaroni/spaghetti, pastries, candies, cookies, pop, and commercial cereals are all devoid of it. Since these "foods" constitute a significant percentage of the calories consumed by America's children, virtually all such children are severely deficient in vitamin E. Exposure for prolonged periods to TVs and video games, as well as to passive smoke from parents who smoke, only deepens the deficiency. As a result, it is easy to comprehend why millions of children develop severe vitamin E deficiencies. Such diets can be easily boosted by using the Pumpkinol on salads, potatoes, vegetables and meats.

Nitrated meats, which are common foods on children's menus (ham, bacon, salami, and bologna are all loaded with nitrates), are significant vitamin E destroyers.   Children usually prefer these meats to fresh meats and fish, such as organ meats, beef, lamb, or salmon, all of which contain significant amounts of vitamin E. The consumption of empty-nutrient foods, such as juices, pop, pastries, cookies, and candy, instead of fresh fruits and vegetables further potentiates the deficiency. What's more, the foods children typically eat are loaded with deep fried oils, margarine, and hydrogenated oils, all of which destroy this vitamin. Add to this the fact that inorganic iron, which is found in all white flour products, oxidizes vitamin E, and it becomes readily understood why nearly all non-supplemented American children are deficient in this nutrient.

VITAMIN E TEST (each response worth 1 point)

Which of these apply to you ?

1. cold hands and/or feet
2. tendency to form blood clots
3. easy bruising
4. swollen legs and/or ankles
5. varicose veins
6. leg and/or foot cramps
7. infertility
8. impotence
9. liver spots (brown spots on the skin)
10. muscular wasting
11. intolerance to dietary oils
12. cataracts and/or macular degeneration
13. Do you have liver disease?
14. Do you consume alcohol on a daily basis?
15. Do you consume foods containing white flour on a daily basis?
16. Do you consume deep fried foods on a daily or weekly basis?
17. Do you use margarine as a spread, or do you use margarine/shortening in cooking?
18. Do you cook with refined vegetable oils such as Crisco oil, Canola oil, sunflower oil, peanut oil, or "light" olive oil?
19. Are you chronically exposed to radioactivity (nuclear plant workers, x-ray technicians, computer programmers, policemen, etc.)?
20. Do you drink fluoridated and/or chlorinated water?
21. Are you taking cholesterol-lowering medications such as Mevacor, Pravachol, Lopid, Lipitor, or Questran?
22. Are you taking iron supplements or multiple vitamin-mineral tablets containing iron?

23. Do you have a history of heart disease and/or angina?
24. Do you tear or injure your muscles or joints easily?
25. Do you consume snack foods, such as chips, pastries, candy bars, pretzels, popcorn, pop, cookies, etc., on a regular basis?
26. Do you have a history of chronic circulatory disease such as Raynaud's syndrome, vasculitis, atherosclerosis, or coronary arterial occlusion?
27. Do you have a history of Peyronie's disease (i.e. erection which fails to recede)?
28. Do you have hemolytic anemia and/or sickle cell anemia?
29. Have you had repeated miscarriages?
30. Do you have chronic obstructive lung disease, particularly emphysema?
31. Are you exposed to heavy air pollution?
32. Are you undergoing chemotherapy/radiation treatments?
33. Do you suffer from hot flashes?
34. Do you have fibrocystic breast disease?
34. Is your skin highly sensitive to sunlight?

Your Score _____

---

1 to 10 points *Mild vitamin E deficiency*: Take 400 I.U. of vitamin E daily. Eat a handful of raw sunflower seeds every day. Increase the consumption of dark green leafy vegetables. Use pure hazelnut or pumpkinseed oil on salads.

11 to 21 points *Moderate vitamin E deficiency*: Take 800 to 1200 I.U. of vitamin E daily. Eat raw sunflower seeds or almonds on a daily basis, along with other foods rich in vitamin E. Also, as a full spectrum natural vitamin E source take crude fortified pumpkinseed oil (i.e. Pumpkinol), 3 tablespoons daily. This tasty oil is super-rich in natural vitamin E and contains the full spectrum of this vitamin. Pumpkinol is stabilized, which prevents the vitamin E from oxidizing. It is the ideal vitamin E source for those allergic to soybeans, from which most commercial vitamin E is derived.

22 and above *Severe vitamin E deficiency*: Warning—severe vitamin E deficiency increases the risks for a variety of illnesses, including heart disease, hardening of the arteries, lupus, Parkinson's disease, anemia, infertility, and immune deficiency. Take 1200 to 1600 I.U. of vitamin E on a daily basis. An example of a vitamin E-rich snack would be two handfuls of raw sunflower seeds or hazelnuts daily. Eat a large salad made with dark greens and topped with chopped raw almonds, hazelnuts, or sunflower seeds every day. Also, take Pumpkinol (crude Austrian pumpkin-seed oil), 4 tablespoons daily, either straight, in juice, or on salads. This is a top natural source of vitamin E. If you are allergic to soy, the source of vitamin E, the fortified and naturally stabilized Pumpkinol is ideal. It is also the ideal vitamin E source for children as well as breast feeding mothers. This is a completely natural source of vitamin E versus the type commonly available, which is from genetically-engineered soybeans.

Vitamin K

Vitamin K is essential to our very survival. That is because there is a function dependent upon vitamin K without which life could not exist, not even for a second: blood clotting. Vitamin K controls this life or death function by stimulating the synthesis of blood-clotting factors in the liver.

Henrik Dam of Denmark discovered this nutrient and indirectly gave it its name, the initial "K" being derived from the Danish word "koagulation". His fascinating research documented how animals fed low-fat diets developed internal bleeding and thinning of the blood. In 1935 Dam provided final proof that vitamin K, a component of fatty foods, is essential for the maintenance of normal blood clotting.

Severe vitamin K deficiency is potentially life-threatening, although such extreme reductions in vitamin K levels are relatively rare. However, that is only because the human body has a stop-gap; it can synthesize enough vitamin K on a daily basis to keep blood clotting normalized. Vitamin K is synthesized in the liver but is also produced by certain naturally occurring intestinal organisms. The intestinal organisms are of such major importance in the synthesis of vitamin K that a disruption in their integrity readily leads to a deficiency. According to Robbin's *Pathological Basis of Disease* intestinal bacterial synthesis is "the most important source" of vitamin K. Thus, drugs which alter or destroy the intestinal bacterial flora, such as antibiotics and cortisone, are a primary cause of vitamin K deficiency.

Recent research has delineated the importance of dietary intake for maintaining optimal vitamin K status. Top food sources include alfalfa meal, spinach, Brussels sprouts, cabbage, cauliflower, kale, liver, and lean meats.

VITAMIN K TEST

Which of these apply to you (each response worth 1 point)?

1. easy bruising
2. bleeding gums
3. spontaneous hemorrhaging (bleeding from the ears, nose, or rectum, etc.)
4. petechiae (tiny blood spots on the skin)
5. bone loss and/or frequent fractures
6. poorly formed (sloppy) stools
7. intermittent and/or chronic diarrhea
8. Have you taken numerous dosages of antibiotics in the past?
9. Do you have a history of repeated miscarriages?
10. Do you avoid eating dark green leafy vegetables?
11. Have you had a portion of your small intestines or colon removed?
12. Do you consume chlorinated water?
13. Do you avoid eating red meats and/or organ meats?

14. Are you on a low cholesterol diet and/or are you taking cholesterol-lowering medications?
15. Do you have intestinal parasitic infection?
16. Do you have chronic candidiasis (i.e. chronic yeast infection)?
17. Are you on Coumadin or Heparin therapy?
18. Do you suffer from Crohn's disease, irritable bowel syndrome, dumping syndrome, or ulcerative colitis?
19. Do you take birth control pills on a regular basis, or have you in the past taken them over a prolonged time?
20. Are you currently taking antibiotics on a daily or weekly basis?
21. Do you have pancreatic and/or liver disease?
22. Do you consume alcoholic beverages on a daily basis?
23. Do you suffer from gallbladder attacks, or do you have gallstones?
24. Has your gallbladder been removed?
25. Do you suffer from gluten intolerance (celiac disease)?
26. Do your peripheral blood vessels burst easily?
27. Do you have a significant family history of stroke, or have you suffered a stroke?
28. Do you have spider or varicose veins?
29. Do you suffer from osteoporosis (thinning of the bones)?
30. Do you take mineral oil or castor oil on a regular basis?

Your Score ____

1 to 6 points *Mild vitamin K deficiency*: At this level correction should be readily achieved through dietary measures. Increase the intake of dark green leafy vegetables and take alfalfa leaf meal as a daily nutritional supplement.

7 to 15 points *Moderate vitamin K deficiency*: Take a multiple vitamin tablet containing vitamin K plus take alfalfa leaf powder on a daily basis. Consume hefty helpings of raw dark greens every day. Take an acidophilus supplement on a daily basis and avoid consumption of all antibiotics. Also, as a crude natural source of vitamin K take Gene's Greens, 2 to 3 dropperfuls daily.

16 and above *Severe vitamin K deficiency*: If you are suffering from repeated episodes of bleeding, see your doctor immediately. Stop taking aspirin, cholesterol-lowering medicines, blood thinners, and antibiotics at once, since these drugs destroy vitamin K. Take a multiple vitamin containing vitamin K on a daily basis. In addition, take 1200 I.U. of vitamin E daily, since it helps conserve and regenerate vitamin K. Vitamin C and bioflavonoid supplements may also be beneficial, since they help keep arterial tissues strong and prevent bleeding. Most importantly, check with your health food store to see if natural vitamin K supplements are available. If so, take 2 or more capsules daily for at least 60 days. Also, take a crude natural source of vegetable-based vitamin K, i.e. Gene's Wild Greens, 4 droppersful daily. The Gene's Greens is only available by mail order: 1-800-243-5242. Consume friendly bacteria supplements daily with meals to reestablish bacterial flora in the gut. Avoid commercial meats, since they contain residues of antibiotics.

Calcium

Undoubtedly, calcium is the most well-known mineral and also the one most commonly taken as a supplement. Millions of women consume it with the hope of preventing bone loss. However, calcium has numerous additional uses as a nutritional supplement. It seems that every week this mineral makes the headlines regarding its importance in human nutrition. This is rightfully so, since every cell in the human body needs it to survive.

While too much calcium can be dangerous, usually the problem is that people fail to get enough. Millions of Americans are suffering from the ill effects of calcium deficiency. The most vulnerable populations are adolescents and the elderly. However, deficiency in children is also common. A wide range of disorders may result, including attention deficit, growth retardation, tooth formation, leg cramps, nosebleed, and bone deformities.

Calcium is the most abundant mineral in the body, some 99% of it being found in the bones. Thus, the bones serve as the calcium reservoir. If there is too much calcium, the body deposits it in the bones. On the other hand, if individuals become deficient in calcium, the bones release it into the blood. This protective mechanism is necessary, because without calcium certain critical organ systems, such as the nervous system, heart, and arteries, would degenerate and death could result. Fortunately, calcium deficiency of this extreme occurs only rarely in the United States.

Since calcium deficiency occurs primarily at the expense of the skeleton, a number of symptoms specifically related to the bones and joints may result. However, because this mineral also controls the function of the nerves, an endless list of musculoskeletal and neurological symptoms may develop as a result of mild to moderate calcium deficiency.

Severe calcium deficiency occurs most commonly in certain high risk groups. These groups include diabetics, cardiac patients, post-surgical patients, elderly individuals, Alzheimer's and Parkinson's patients, arthritis sufferers, and nursing home occupants. Additionally, certain substances antagonize calcium absorption and/or cause calcium loss into the urine or stool. These substances include:

aspirin	tetracycline
cortisone	calcium-channel blockers
chemotherapeutic agents	antacids

Cortisone is one of the chief calcium antagonizing drugs, since it causes massive mobilization of calcium from bone. With cortisone therapy, the calcium losses may be so severe that the entire skeleton becomes porous. In fact, the bones may become so weak that they split or crack spontaneously. In addition, people who fail to exercise regularly are at high risk for osteoporosis. Sleeping on a soft mattress also increases the risk.

Calcium absorption is dependent upon vitamin D. This vitamin can be consumed through the diet, but it is also synthesized in the skin, a reaction which requires sunlight. Thus, those who live in regions with short summers and/or people who rarely go outdoors are likely to be calcium deficient. Additionally, bedridden and wheelchair-bound patients usually develop rather severe calcium deficiencies. This category includes nursing home occupants as well as the thousands of bedfast individuals who occupy the hospitals. The risk factors for such individuals are extensive and are listed as follows:

a) they are usually taking drugs which impair calcium absorption.

b) they get little or no exercise and, thus, readily lose calcium from their bones.

c) they spend most of their time in bed.

d) they get little or no sunlight.

e) they usually receive less than the RDA for calcium and vitamin D in their diets.

f) their diets are high in refined sugars, which disrupt calcium metabolism and cause bone loss.

g) they absorb calcium poorly even if taking it supplementally; this is largely due to the decreased production of stomach acid that invariably occurs in poorly nourished and/or elderly individuals; hydrochloric acid is essential for calcium digestion and assimilation.

h) they receive little or no food rich in vitamin A, a nutrient required for efficient calcium absorption and transport.

It is no surprise that spontaneous fractures of the hips and/or spine are a prime cause of morbidity and mortality in the elderly. There is a virtual epidemic of calcium and vitamin D deficiency in this population, one that cannot be corrected simply by drinking a glass or two of milk per day. These individuals require the daily intake of absorbable calcium supplements and vitamin D. However, calcium alone is insufficient. The fact is vitamin D plays a greater role in strengthening the bones than calcium, magnesium, and all other minerals combined.

CALCIUM TEST

Which of these apply to you (each response worth 1 point)?

1. joint pain
2. slow pulse rate
3. nervousness or irritability
4. tremors
5. twitching muscles and/or leg cramps
6. anxiety
7. chronic back and/or hip pain
8. vulnerability to fractures
9. loose teeth
10. tendency to form cavities
11. brittle nails
12. high blood pressure
13. numbness and/or tingling of the extremities
14. spastic stomach
15. muscular tension or tight, spastic muscles
16. chronic headaches
17. soft teeth
18. vertically ridged nails
19. Do you get little or no exposure to sunshine?
20. Do you have irritable bowel syndrome (colitis)?
21. Do you avoid eating fresh fish and/or milk products?
22. Do you drink three or more cups of coffee per day?
23. Are you a cigarette, pipe, or cigar smoker?
24. Do you regularly take cortisone or use cortisone creams?

25. Do you regularly consume antacids?
26. Do you regularly take tetracycline?
27. Are you on calcium channel blockers?
28. Have you undergone or are you currently undergoing chemotherapy?
29. Do you get little or no exercise?
30. Are you currently bedridden and/or wheelchair-bound?
31. Do you consume refined sugar on a daily basis?

Your Score ____

---

1 to 9 points *Mild calcium deficiency*: A mild calcium deficit is easily corrected by increasing the consumption of calcium-rich foods. Try the Calcium-Rich Vegetable Juice Cocktail listed in the recipe section. Eat foods rich in vitamin D for aiding calcium absorption. If you can tolerate milk products, eat two cups of yogurt or cottage cheese daily. In addition, be sure to exercise regularly, since physical activity aids in the deposition of calcium into bone. Supplementation may be indicated; calcium has a calming effect upon the nervous system. Furthermore, it is protective against cancer of the colon. Calcium absorption is best when supplements are taken at bedtime.

10 to 19 points *Moderate calcium deficiency*: Follow all the recommendations for mild calcium deficiency. In addition, to further enhance absorption take a multiple vitamin containing vitamin D and calcium along with an additional 500 mg of supplemental calcium. Walk one mile or more every day. For best absorption take supplemental calcium at bedtime, using calcium with vitamin C or lemon juice. Avoid substances which deplete tissue calcium: cigarette smoke, coffee, antacids, cortisone, soda pop, and refined sugars. As a natural source of calcium take crude wild oregano capsules, (i.e. OregaMax} six daily. Calcium absorption is best when supplements are taken at bedtime.

20 or above *Severe calcium deficiency*: This level of deficiency may not be entirely the result of a calcium-deficient diet. Numerous disease processes may induce severe calcium deficit. Included are chronic kidney infections and other renal diseases, hyperparathyroidism, hyperthyroidism, hepatitis, cirrhosis of the liver, sluggish liver syndrome, and cancer. Notice the emphasis upon liver disorders; that is because this organ synthesizes calcium-binding proteins, without which this mineral cannot be absorbed. Additionally, vitamin D deficiency may cause calcium loss, even if the dietary intake of this mineral is adequate. To correct the calcium deficit, follow the aforementioned advice. In addition, take 1000 to 1500 mg of absorbable calcium daily. Avoid oyster shell calcium. This type of supplement is poorly absorbed, and its consumption has been linked to kidney stone formation. Another form to avoid is bone meal, or ground bone, since it usually contains residues of heavy metals, particularly lead. Calcium citrate, hydroxyapatite, or calcium lactate would be preferable. Additionally, increase the intake of calcium-rich foods and drink the Calcium-Rich Vegetable Juice Cocktail daily (see recipe in Appendix B). Be sure to increase your fluid intake when taking large doses of calcium. Walk two or more miles per day and/or be sure to partake in other exercises regularly in order to stimulate calcium deposition into bone. As a natural source of highly absorbable calcium take crude wild oregano capsules, (i.e. OregaMax) 4 twice daily. Calcium absorption is best when supplements are taken at bedtime.

Chromium

Chromium is perhaps best known as chrome, which is the metallic form of this mineral. Chrome obviously has no nutritional value. Yet, organic chromium, the type found in food, is absorbed and utilized by the body.

Chromium is essential for the function of the blood sugar regulating system. It aids in the absorption of sugar into the bloodstream and helps drive sugar in the form of glucose into the cells so it can be utilized as fuel. Additionally, chromium is involved in the digestion and metabolism of fats and proteins.

Chromium deficiency is common in the United States. This is largely a consequence of the refinement of foods, particularly grains, a process which results in the destruction of virtually all of the naturally occurring chromium. For instance, whole-grain wheat, rye, and barley are excellent sources of chromium, but when these grains are refined into flour, chromium losses may reach 95%.

Determining if an individual is chromium deficient through medical testing isn't easy. The deficiency simply must be presumed, since the American diet is devoid of it. A study by the U.S. Department of Agriculture found that the diets of 90% of Americans tested were deficient in chromium. This is certainly due to a lack of it in the diet but is also a result of the consumption of chromium-depleting agents, particularly refined sugars. An additional factor is stress, which causes a loss of this mineral into urine and/or stool. Physical stress may wreak more havoc on chromium stores than even mental stress. The results of one study appearing in *Sports Medicine* (1987) showed that the urine of joggers completing a six mile run contained five times the normal amount of chromium.

Chromium is involved in the metabolism of fats and sugars. A lack of it results in the distorted function of insulin, the hormone that regulates blood sugar levels. In fact, chromium deficiency can ultimately lead to an insulin deficiency in addition to reducing insulin's effectiveness. The result is blood sugar disturbances, elevated blood fats, high blood sugar, and, ultimately, diabetes.

Chromium is found in relatively few foods. Fruits and vegetables contain virtually none, and most processed foods are devoid of it. Top sources include brewer's yeast, whole grains, rice polishings (Nutri-Sense), eggs, crude red grape powder, and black pepper. The red grape powder is available as a supplement, i.e. Resvitanol powder. This is the top naturally occurring source of chromium. Incredibly, a large heaping teaspoon contains nearly half the RDA.

CHROMIUM TEST

Which of these apply to you (each response worth 1 point)?

1. blood sugar disturbances
2. difficulty losing weight
3. chronic fatigue
4. intolerance to sugar or starch
5. tendency to rapidly gain weight after eating sugars and/or starches
6. cravings for sugars and/or starches
7. poor muscle tone and/or muscular weakness
8. chronic or morbid obesity
9. chronic depression and/or anxiety
10. craving for sweets, especially after meals
11. sudden loss of weight
12. episodes of shakiness
13. reversible tremors
14. Do you have a history of infertility and/or reduced sperm count?
15. Do you have high blood cholesterol levels?
16. Do you have high blood triglyceride levels?
17. Do you have elevated blood sugar and/or diabetes?
18. Do you consume refined sugar, as hidden sugar in foods or beverages, on a daily basis?
19. Do you regularly consume alcoholic beverages (4 or more drinks per week)?
20. Do you regularly consume white flour products such as white bread, buns, muffins, toast, pasta, crackers, or doughnuts?
21. On average, do you jog 2 or more miles every day?
22. Do you fall asleep after eating starchy or sugary foods?
23. Do you eat white rice on a regular basis?
24. Do you have a history of cataracts or macular degeneration?
25. Do you have a history of arterial blockage, hardening of the arteries, or coronary artery disease?

26. Are you nearsighted?
27. Do you have blurry vision?

Your Score _____

---

1 to 6 points *Mild chromium deficiency*: Increase your consumption of chromium-rich foods, reduce your sugar and alcohol intake, and take 100 mcg of chromium, preferably as picolinate or GTF (i.e. glucose tolerance factor), twice daily.

7 to 12 points *Moderate chromium deficiency*: At this level tissue damage is likely to occur as a result of impaired sugar and/or fat metabolism. In particular, chromium deficiency has been associated with degeneration of the arteries. Obesity is also a probable result of a moderate deficiency. Take 200 mcg of chromium two or three times daily, and reduce the intake of white sugar, flour, and rice. Avoid alcoholic beverages and sugar-sweetened drinks. Take 3 heaping tablespoons of rice polishings or Nutri-Sense daily mixed in juice, water, or milk. Also, take crude red grape powder, a top source of natural chromium, two heaping teaspoons daily (if taking capsules, 3 to 4 caps twice daily). Also, as a natural source of chromium take crude red grape powder, that is Resvitanol, four capsules twice daily. This provides a highly usable natural type of chromium.

13 to 19 points *Severe chromium deficiency*: Warning—if tissue damage is imminent the chromium deficiency remains unresolved. Hypoglycemia, diabetes, morbid obesity, cataracts, depression, anxiety, cancer, and/or heart disease all are likely to result. Eliminate dietary sources of refined sugar and curtail the intake of alcoholic beverages. Foods containing white flour or rice should also be eliminated from the diet. Take 250 mcg of chromium three times daily. In addition, consume 3 heaping tablespoons of rice polishings or Nutri-Sense morning and night mixed in water, milk, or juice. Add Nutri-Sense to the diet whenever possible as an additive to cereals and/or recipes. Try the Chromium Shake in the recipe section of this book. Also, take crude red grape powder, 3 heaping teaspoons daily. This is a top source of naturally occurring chromium. A large heaping teaspoon contains nearly 50% of the minimum daily requirement of this nutrient. Also, as a natural source of chromium take Resvitanol, four capsules twice daily. This provides a highly usable natural type of chromium.

20 and above *Extreme chromium deficiency*: Warning—tissue damage is imminent if the chromium deficiency remains unresolved. Hypoglycemia, diabetes, morbid obesity, cataracts, depression, anxiety, cancer, and/or heart disease all are likely to result. Eliminate dietary sources of refined sugar and curtail the intake of alcoholic beverages. Foods containing white flour or rice should also be eliminated from the diet. Take 500 mcg of chromium three times daily. In addition, consume 3 heaping tablespoons of Nutri-Sense morning and night mixed in water, milk, or juice. Add Nutri-Sense to the diet whenever possible as an additive to cereals and/or recipes. Try the Chromium Shake in the recipe section of this book. Also, take crude red grape powder, 3 heaping teaspoons daily. This is a top source of naturally occurring chromium. A large heaping teaspoon contains nearly 50% of the minimum daily requirement of this nutrient. Also, as a natural source of chromium take crude red grape powder, that is Resvitanol, four capsules three times daily or if using the powder, a heaping teaspoon three times daily. This provides a highly usable natural type of chromium.

Copper

The first evidence for the essential nature of copper in human nutrition was discovered in 1928. A lack of it led to anemia in all subjects tested. Today, copper deficiency is relatively uncommon but only for one reason: copper pipes. Most Americans get their RDA of copper just by drinking tap water. However, not everyone drinks tap water, and not all tap water runs through copper pipes.

Deficiency of copper may occur as a result of a processed food diet. Additionally, certain groups are at an exceptionally high risk for copper deficiency. These groups include:

- those undergoing high-dose zinc therapy
- gastrectomy patients
- those taking multiple medications
- individuals consuming a high sugar diet
- cancer patients undergoing chemotherapy
- patients with chronic liver disease, including cirrhosis and hepatitis
- individuals with celiac spine
- individuals who have had a portion of their intestines or stomach removed or stapled

Copper is an essential component of numerous human enzymes, including superoxide dismutase (SOD). Additionally, it works together with iron in the building of red blood cells. Thus, copper is an important anti-anemia factor. It is also involved in the maintenance of the health of arterial tissues, and if copper deficiency becomes extreme, degeneration of the arteries usually results.

For individuals with chronic arthritis, the "copper bracelet" may not be entirely an old wives' tale. This is because joint degeneration has been associated with trace mineral deficiencies, copper being one of them.

Perhaps the most common cause of extreme copper deficiency is the consumption of excessive amounts of refined sugar. In addition to being deficient in copper, sugar causes the loss of this nutrient into the stool and urine. Another common cause of extreme copper deficiency is megadose zinc therapy. This is because zinc impedes the absorption of copper. Usually, dosages of 90 mg or more per day are required to artificially induce copper deficit. Anyone consuming large amounts of zinc should supplement their diet with copper. Top food sources of copper include rice bran, liver, red meats, whole grains, and mushrooms.

COPPER TEST

Which of these apply to you (each response worth 1 point)?

1. heart rhythm disturbances
2. alopecia (patchy hair loss)
3. skin rashes
4. diarrhea
5. fatigue
6. fragile or brittle bones
7. difficulty breathing
8. anemia
9. infertility
10. numbness or paresthesia
11. bitter taste in the mouth
12. poor wound healing
13. delayed healing of fractures or sprains
14. Are you a diabetic?
15. Do you have a significant family history of diabetes?
16. Do you suffer from hardening of the arteries?
17. Do you consume sugar, particularly fructose, regularly?
18. Do you have a high cholesterol level?
19. Do you have osteoarthritis?
20. Do you take 75 mg or more of zinc daily?
21. Do you perspire heavily?
22. Do you eat primarily processed foods?

Your Score ____

1 to 5 points *Mild copper deficiency*: Take a multiple-vitamin tablet containing copper and increase the consumption of foods rich in copper. Avoid all sources of refined sugar.

6 to 11 points *Moderate copper deficiency*: Take 4 mg of copper daily. Include large helpings of copper-rich foods in the diet. Avoid refined sugars and reduce the consumption of alcohol. Take Chelated copper, 2 to 4 milligrams daily.

12 and above *Severe copper deficiency*: Take 4 to 6 mg of Chelated copper twice daily. Eat copper rich foods on a daily basis; rice bran or polishings, liver, and (organic) soy products, are excellent sources. Curtail the consumption of refined sugars, particularly fructose, which is specific for inducing copper deficiency.

Iodine

It was nearly sixty years ago that iodine made global news as a miracle cure. Singlehandedly, it eliminated a disfiguring and potentially life-threatening disease: goiter. This is because iodine is an essential component of thyroid hormone.

The goiter belt of the United States includes primarily the states surrounding the Great Lakes: Wisconsin, Illinois, Michigan, Ohio, and Indiana. Prior to the introduction of iodized salt, goiter was endemic in these regions. Several Canadian provinces, particularly Ontario, Manitoba, and Quebec, are also a part of the goiter belt. All these regions have one thing in common; they have little or no iodine in their soils. Thus, food grown in these regions was and still is devoid of iodine. For some people this may not pose a problem, that is if the individuals are consuming sufficient amounts of iodine in the form of iodized salt, sea salt, or foods naturally rich in iodine. Unfortunately, many people living in the goiter belt are placed on salt-restricted diets for health reasons. These patients are often under the care of dietitians, who painstakingly eliminate all traces of salt from their diets and, thus, artificially induce an iodine deficiency. Unless such individuals are consuming significant amounts of fish and/or seafood rich in iodine, a severe iodine deficiency usually results.

Patients placed on salt-restricted diets who fail to consume iodine-rich foods are highly vulnerable to the development of goiter and other iodine-deficiency diseases. Many of these individuals rarely eat seafood. Therefore, iodine deficiency is common and so are the diseases it induces: hypothyroidism (underactive thyroid), hyperthyroidism (overactive thyroid), and goiter.

In some areas the medical profession appears to have reverted to the Dark Ages, prescribing all manner of highly toxic substances for the treatment of disease. Radioactive iodine is a favorite noxious agent for the treatment of overactive thyroid. It is used to destroy thyroid cells. This method of treatment is based upon the belief that if the thyroid gland is overactive, it must be destroyed before it destroys the patient. Just why the thyroid gland is operating out of control is rarely investigated. No consideration is given to the fact that as early as the 1930s, hyperthyroidism was proven to result simply from nutritional deficiency, with a lack of iodine heading the list. Unfortunately, the ultimate result of contaminating the thyroid with radioactive iodine is to create a physician-induced and permanent case of under-active thyroid, forcing the patient to become dependent upon thyroid medication for life. Yet, the problem could have been quickly resolved if the iodine deficiency, as well as the other nutritional deficits which caused malfunction of the thyroid gland, would have been judiciously corrected. Thyroid-nourishing nutrients include:

potassium	pantothenic acid
tyrosine	niacin
magnesium	folic acid
vitamin C	coenzyme Q-1O
thiamine	zinc
riboflavin	copper

What a crime it is that many a thyroid has been destroyed by radioactive iodine and/or other potent chemicals when a half pound of shrimp per day along with a few nutritional supplements would have entirely resolved the problem.

On the negative side iodine is perhaps the most allergenic of all minerals. Allergic reactions to iodine can be quite severe. Perhaps the most commonly occurring reaction is to radioactive iodine, which is the type used in electronic medical imaging as well as x-ray diagnosis and treatment. The iodine is utilized as a carrier medium for a radioactive tracer, which concentrates in the thyroid. With thyroid studies, a bolus of radioactive iodine is injected into the veins.

Some of this iodine is excreted via the urine. However, the thyroid gland aggressively concentrates the remaining radioactive iodine from the blood. In cases of goiter, thyroid nodules, hyperthyroidism, or other inflammatory thyroid diseases, medical specialists detect large concentrations of iodine in the x-rays. Other tests in which radioactive contrast media are used include cat scans, bone scans, and thallium heart scans.

Iodine allergies/reactions can also occur with the ingestion of dietary sources, including iodized salt, iodine-rich foods, and iodine supplements. A common reaction to iodine is acne outbreaks. However, reactions may be of a far more severe nature and may include asthmatic attacks, hives or other rashes, throat closure, shock, and even death. One way to neutralize iodine reactions is to take a high-quality edible wild oregano extract, for instance, Oreganol. To prevent iodine reactions take 2 to 3 drops twice daily or one gelcap twice daily. Oreganol may also be taken to reverse acute iodine reactions.

Iodine's most celebrated function relates to its role in thyroid gland metabolism. Simply put, the synthesis of thyroid hormone is entirely dependent upon it, and this explains why nearly all the body's iodine is concentrated in the thyroid gland.

When ingested, iodine exerts an antibiotic-like action. Studies have shown that white blood cells absorb iodine from the blood and use it to enhance their microbial killing capacities. This mineral serves an additional valuable function related to immune function: it prevents mucous buildup. It seems that iodine is necessary to keep the mucous that lines many of the internal organs fluid or thin. This is especially valuable for individuals suffering from lung diseases such as emphysema, chronic bronchitis, pneumonia, asthma, and/or cystic fibrosis. Top food sources of iodine include unprocessed sea salt, shrimp, crab, lobster, sea fish, seaweed, and cattle/fowl raised on iodine-rich feed.

IODINE TEST

Which of these apply to you (each response worth 1 point)?

1. cystic and/or sore ovaries
2. cystic breast disease
3. severe menstrual cramps
4. heavy menstrual bleeding
5. heightened susceptibility to infectious disease, especially bronchitis, pneumonia, ear infections, and/or strep throat
6. chronic fatigue or lethargy
7. morning fatigue improving as the day proceeds
8. chronic skin infections (boils, acne, fungal infections, etc.)
9. excess mucous and/or thick mucous in the throat
10. stuffy sinuses
11. cold extremities/highly sensitive to cold weather
12. muscular fatigue and/or cramps
13. stunted growth
14. coarse hair
15. reduced body temperature
16. mental sluggishness
17. Do you have an overactive or underactive thyroid?
18. Are you on a low sodium diet?
19. Do you avoid consuming fish or sea food?
20. Do you have a low libido (sluggish sex drive)?
21. Do you have a history of goiter?

22. Are you 20 or more pounds overweight and/or do you have a difficult time losing weight?
23. Are you a night owl?
24. Are you a total vegetarian?
25. Do you have a history of infertility and/or low sperm count?
26. Do you have cellulite?
27. Do you have high cholesterol, above 220?

Your Score ____

---

1 to 6 points *Mild iodine deficiency:* Increase the consumption of iodine-rich foods. Use crude sea salt in all recipes. As a natural supplemental source of kelp take Thyronorm, two capsules daily.

7 to 14 points *Moderate iodine deficiency:* Iodine deficiency impairs thyroid function and weakens immunity. Eat iodine-rich fish and seafood. As a natural source of iodine, take Thyronorm, four capsules daily. Use sea salt with all meals and recipes.

15 and above *Severe iodine deficiency:* Crab, lobster, salmon, cod, mackerel, halibut, and shrimp should be regular items in your diet. However, try to purchase seafood from areas with reduced pollution such as Alaskan and Icelandic waters[7]. Add seaweed and/or kelp[8] to your salads and soups. As a natural

---

7. Seafood from contaminated waters is a health risk for several reasons: contamination by chemicals, radioactive material, heavy metals, and human waste (sewage). Recently a rash of cases of food poisonings have occurred from consuming shellfish contaminated by such organisms as Salmonella, E. coli, and even cholera. If you consume seafood, rinse with large amounts of water, cook it thoroughly, and never eat it raw.

8. Recently, researchers have discovered that kelp from polluted waters is contaminated with heavy metals, particularly arsenic. In fact, certain individuals consuming kelp developed arsenic toxicity. Use kelp only if it is harvested from a region of low pollution. Note: ThyroNorm, rich in wild kelp, is free of such contaminants.

126 Nutrition Tests for Better Health

source of toxin-free kelp take ThyroNorm, four capsules twice daily. Use sea salt with all foods. Additionally, be sure to avoid the iodine antagonists. These substances, known medically as goitrogens, are found in certain foods, notably Brussels sprouts, soybeans, almonds, rapeseed, beans, peanuts, cabbage, spinach, turnips, carrots (and carrot juice), beets, broccoli, cauliflower, peaches, pears, flax, and kale. However, cooking inactivates the iodine antagonists and, thus, only the raw forms of these foods must be avoided. There is a word of caution. Certain individuals are highly sensitive to iodine. This sensitivity can result in potentially life-threatening allergic reactions. If you develop any unusual symptoms after increasing your iodine intake, stop consuming the iodine immediately. In any case, if you rarely consume seafood and do not take supplemental iodine, be sure to introduce the iodine slowly. Despite these precautions, iodine is a natural substance and is well tolerated by the majority of individuals.

Iron

Iron is one of the few nutrients that is a two-edged sword; it can be life-threatening to have either too little or too much of it. Most people are aware of the primary result of too little iron—Geritol commercials took care of that. However, there is a paucity of literature concerning the dangers of iron excess. A little known fact is that iron toxicity is a major cause of poisoning in children (from overdosing on vitamin tablets containing iron). In addition, excess iron is a predisposing factor for a variety of degenerative diseases, including cancer, arthritis, heart disease, Alzheimer's disease, and liver disease. The excess iron accumulates within certain organs, causing cellular damage and even cell death. If cell death is extensive, organ failure can occur, which may result in fatality. Organs wherein iron readily accumulates include the bone marrow, spleen, liver, kidneys, lungs, brain, and heart.

In extreme cases of iron overload the excess iron is deposited in every organ, in fact, in every cell of the body. This condition is known as *hemochromatosis*. A similar condition, *hemosiderosis*, is less severe but may proceed to hemochromatosis, the latter being usually fatal. If caught in the early stages, patients with hemosiderosis can be cured by a combination of several therapies. Most important is eliminating all sources of dietary and supplemental iron. Additionally, physicians often prescribe phlebotomy, or bloodletting, as a means of lowering iron stores. Iron chelating agents, that is compounds which bind and remove iron from the tissues, may also be prescribed.

Due to the dangers of iron overload vitamins containing iron should be avoided except by those who are diagnosed with iron deficiency. Pregnant, breast-feeding, and menstruating women may also need additional iron. Men should never take supplemental iron unless under a physician's care for iron deficiency diseases. Iron-free multiple vitamin and mineral tablets are now available at many health food stores.

Iron is one of the largest minerals, molecularly. Thus, it may be difficult to absorb. The addition of acidic substances to the diet, such as tomato sauce, lemon juice, vinegar and citric acid, greatly enhances absorption. Additionally, vitamin C potentiates the absorption of iron. Top dietary sources of iron include organ meats, red meats, blackstrap molasses, oysters, almonds, cocoa powder, caviar, pistachios, and dark green leafy vegetables.

IRON TEST

Which of these apply to you (each response worth 1 point)?

1. chronic fatigue
2. lack of appetite
3. spoon shaped (scooped) nails
4. confusion
5. memory loss
6. lightheadedness or dizziness
7. rapid heartbeat after minimal exercise
8. inflamed and/or sore tongue

  9. irritability
 10. chronic headaches
 11. fragile bones
 12. difficulty swallowing
 13. brittle hair and/or nails
 14. depression
 15. constipation
 16. paleness of the skin, especially facial skin
 17. sensitivity to cold
 18. shortness of breath
 19. tingling of the fingers or toes
 20. sores on the inside of or around the mouth
 21. vertical ridges on the fingernails
 22. hair loss, especially in females
 23. cravings for cold water and/or ice (chewing of ice)
 24. Do you take antacids on a regular basis?
 25. Do you drink three or more cups of black or green tea on a daily basis?
 26. Do you have rheumatoid arthritis?
 27. Are you anemic?
 28. Have you suffered from heavy menstrual flow for a prolonged time span?
 29. Do you take aspirin and/or non-steroidal anti-inflammatory drugs (i.e., Naprosyn, Indocin, Clinoril, etc.) on a daily basis?

Your Score _____

1 to 6 points *Marginal or no iron deficiency*: Many of the symptoms of iron deficiency are vague and, therefore, may be mimicked by other conditions. Always remember that iron deficiency is best confirmed by blood tests. Do not take large amounts of synthetic iron unless you have a blood-test confirmed iron deficiency.

7 to 12 points *Mild iron deficiency*: Never take supplemental iron on the basis of a symptom quiz only. If you are concerned about being iron deficient, see your doctor and attempt confirmation through blood testing. Such tests should include a serum iron level, iron-binding protein, and a serum ferritin level. Ferritin is a storage form of iron and is an excellent indicator of the total body burden of this nutrient.

13 to 19 points *Moderate iron deficiency*: Follow the aforementioned advice. Blood testing to determine the extent of the deficiency is indicated. Take a multiple vitamin-mineral tablet containing iron (18 mg per day) and increase the consumption of iron-rich foods. Excellent food sources of iron include red meat, liver, egg yolks, dark greens, raisins, and dried apricots. Eat a cup or more of raisins or dried apricots daily.

20 and above *Severe iron deficiency*: At this level of deficiency a measurable decline in red blood cell count, as well as hemoglobin, is likely. Again, blood testing is indicated. If anemia is confirmed (a hemoglobin of less than 13.0 in women and 14.0 in men), take 20 mg of iron as ferrous fumarate or a protein-bound type of iron twice daily. Be sure to take 500 mg of vitamin C with the iron, since it greatly potentiates iron absorption. Additionally, take a multiple vitamin-mineral tablet, 4 mg of copper, and extra B-complex. Organic liver, particularly calves' liver, is an excellent source of natural iron. Eat liver twice weekly, plus consume at least a dozen extra large eggs weekly. Eat a cup or two of raisins or dried apricots daily. Other excellent sources of iron include food extracts such as crude wild oregano capsules (Oregamax) and Resvitanol (crude red grape) powder. The latter are totally natural ways to correct iron deficiency.

Magnesium

In terms of its importance in human nutrition magnesium is one of the most underrated minerals. It is an essential nutrient and is required for the maintenance of some of the most basic functions of life. Crucial organs, such as the heart, brain, and kidneys, are dependent upon it.

A lack of magnesium is associated with a variety of diseases affecting these organs, including coronary artery disease, hardening of the arteries, high blood pressure, heart arrhythmia, kidney stones, kidney infections, pyelonephritis, depression, anxiety, Alzheimer's disease, and Parkinson's disease.

Traditionally, doctors have underestimated the role played by magnesium in the prevention and/or treatment of disease. However, sophisticated blood tests are now proving that magnesium deficiency occurs frequently in the chronically ill. The fact is the deficiency of this mineral in America is so common that it should be considered epidemic.

Literally hundreds of symptoms, illnesses, and diseases may occur as a result of magnesium deficiency. In fact, a greater number of diseases have been correlated with magnesium deficiency than with the deficiency of any other mineral. This wide range of effects is explained by the fact that magnesium is an integral component of every cell in the body. It is second only to potassium as the most abundant intracellular nutrient. The immense value of magnesium in human nutrition is best illustrated by listing the breadth of its functions, which include:

- neurotransmission and neurotransmitter synthesis
- skeletal muscle contraction
- cellular energy production
- hormone and protein synthesis
- digestion of starches and sugars
- sugar and fat metabolism
- white blood cell synthesis and activity
- digestive enzyme synthesis
- arterial wall contraction/relaxation
- stomach acid production
- antibody synthesis
- bowel motility
- intracellular mineral transport

Magnesium is a large atom and, therefore, it may be difficult to assimilate. Furthermore, it is absorbed more readily from food sources than nutritional supplements. Additionally, certain disease states compromise magnesium absorption, including Crohn's disease, malabsorption syndrome, dumping syndrome, ulcerative colitis, irritable bowel syndrome, anorexia/bulimia, hypochlorhydria (low stomach acid), hypothyroidism (underactive thyroid), celiac disease, intestinal parasitism, and intestinal or stomach cancer. Drugs that deplete tissue levels of magnesium include diuretics, cardiac drugs, cortisone, aspirin, and antibiotics. Additionally, both coffee and alcohol aggressively deplete magnesium from the tissues. Top food sources include whole grains, red meats, fish and seafood, poultry, nuts, hot and/or tangy spices, and cocoa. People who ravenously crave chocolate may be magnesium deficient, since cocoa powder is one of the richest magnesium sources known. Unfortunately, chocolate is always combined with sugar, and sugar causes significant magnesium loss from the tissues.

MAGNESIUM TEST

Which of these apply to you (each response worth 1 point)?

1. heart rhythm disturbances (irregular heartbeat)
2. constipation and/or sluggish colon
3. chronic fatigue
4. muscles tear or injure easily
5. muscle cramps (or cramps in the bottom of the feet)
6. depression
7. muscular weakness
8. inability to control bladder
9. night sweats
10. excessive body odor
11. muscle twitching
12. lower or mid-back pain
13. muscular tension or tight muscles

14. dizziness
15. enlarged facial pores
16. uncontrollable sweating of the hands, feet, and/or armpits
17. painful menstrual cramps
18. PMS
19. restless leg syndrome (i.e. constant jerking or motion of the legs at night)
20. chronic knee and/or hip pain
21. cold hands and/or feet
22. lack of appetite
23. sudden episodes of loss of brain function (mesmerized)
24. nausea
25. rapid heartbeat (above 80 beats per minute)
26. carpal tunnel syndrome
27. nervous agitation (inability to relax)
28. repeated tapping of the hands or feet
29. Are you easily disoriented and/or confused?
30. Do you have high blood pressure?
31. Do you have chronic diarrhea or sloppy stools?
32. Are you easily weakened by stress, or are you physically intolerant of stress?
33. Do you have chronic arthritis?
34. Do you have heart disease and/or angina pectoris?
35. Do you suffer from headaches occurring prior to or during your menstrual cycle?
36. Do you have overactive or underactive thyroid function?
37. Do you have osteoporosis?
38. Do your bones fracture easily, or do they fail to heal after fracturing?
39. Do you suffer from epilepsy or convulsions?
40. Do you drink alcohol on a daily basis (add an additional 3 points)?
41. Do you have a history of kidney stones? (add an additional 2 points)
42. Do you suffer from chronic kidney disease?
43. Do you regularly take diuretic drugs? (add 2 points)

44. Are you a sugar addict? (add an additional 3 points)

Your Score _____

---

1 to 6 points *Mild magnesium deficiency*: Take 400 mg of magnesium daily. The recommended type is magnesium taurate or aspartate, a specialized amino acid chelate which offers the best absorption. Avoid magnesium carbonate, oxide, and sulfate, because they are poorly absorbed. Any supplement containing magnesium oxide is poor in quality. Increase the consumption of magnesium-rich foods, particularly dark green leafy vegetables, almonds, seeds, and hot/tangy spices.

7 to 16 points *Moderate magnesium deficiency*: Follow the aforementioned advice. Also, take 800 mg of an absorbable magnesium daily. Restrict the consumption of refined sugar, white flour, white rice, caffeine, and alcohol. Increase the consumption of magnesium-rich foods, adding them to every meal. As a natural magnesium source take crude wild oregano capsules, i.e. Oregamax, 3 caps twice daily.

17 to 25 points *Severe magnesium deficiency*: A significant decline in tissue levels of magnesium increases the risks for a variety of diseases, including heart disease, arthritis, atherosclerosis, PMS, and high blood pressure. Follow the aforementioned advice. Also, take 900 mg of magnesium daily in a dosage of 300 mg morning, noon, and night. If you are taking diuretics, see your doctor, so he/she can wean you off them. Additionally, alcohol depletes magnesium from the body. Thus, consumption of all alcoholic beverages must be curtailed. Refined sugar also destroys this nutrient. Halt all intake. Consume large helpings of magnesium-rich foods with every meal. Use magnesium-rich spices, such as cumin, basil, and cayenne, in all your cooking. Also take Oregamax, 4 caps twice daily. Caution: If diarrhea occurs as a result of high doses of magnesium, reduce the dose.

26 and above *Extreme magnesium deficiency*: Warning—this level of magnesium deficiency can result in cellular damage in a number of organ systems, including the nerves, bones, joints, heart muscle, brain, kidneys, thyroid glands, and adrenal glands. Follow the aforementioned advice. Also, because of the severity of the deficiency, magnesium injections may be necessary. Even so, it is advisable to take 400 mg of chelated magnesium 3 times daily. There is a word of caution. Magnesium can cause diarrhea. If you develop loose stools, reduce the dosage. Liberally add hot, tangy spices to your foods. Include in your diet Brazil nuts, almonds, cilantro, basil, fennel tea, sage tea, sesame seeds, peanut butter, figs, oatmeal, hazelnuts, and spinach. Also, take Nutri-Sense, which is rich in natural magnesium, 3 or more tablespoons in juice or water daily. Also, take Oregamax, which is the crude wild herb, a natural source of absorbable magnesium, 5 caps twice daily.

Super-High Risk Magnesium Deficiency Test

This test evaluates the risks for diseases of a potentially life-threatening nature that may develop as a consequence of extreme magnesium deficiency. A reduced level of magnesium in the blood or within the cells has been associated with an increased risk for sudden death from heart attacks as well as strokes. Spasm of the coronary arteries, which can result in heart attack, has been proven in numerous scientific studies to be caused by magnesium deficiency. Recent studies document how intravenous infusions of magnesium can reduce the death rate from heart attacks in hospitals by as much as fifty percent. In fact, its value in the treatment of life-threatening cardiovascular disease is so great that researchers are recommending that magnesium infusions be routinely given to all cardiac admissions. The magnesium level within the coronary arteries and/or heart muscle cells is usually severely depressed in heart-attack patients. Thus, magnesium infusions should be available in all ambulances, emergency rooms, and coronary units. There is good reason for this prescription: If the magnesium infusions were given, the need for high-risk invasive procedures, such as cardiac catheterization, coronary angioplasty, and bypass surgery, would be greatly curtailed. Magnesium-deficient individuals also suffer from a heightened incidence of stroke, high blood pressure, dementia, multiple sclerosis, anxiety/depression, Parkinson's disease, and arthritis.

SUPER-HIGH RISK MAGNESIUM DEFICIENCY TEST

Which of these apply to you (each response worth 1 point)?

1. Do you exclusively drink softened, or distilled water (two or more glasses per day)?
2. Do you drink four or more cups of coffee daily?
3. Do you drink four or more cups of hot tea or iced tea daily?
4. Do you consume sweets often?
5. Do you eat refined sugar hidden in foods? (See pages 207-216 for a comprehensive listing of such foods.)
6. Do you eat white flour and white rice products, while avoiding whole grains?
7. Do you drink one or more alcoholic beverages daily (add an additional 3 points if you consume over 4 daily)?
8. Do you smoke 1/2 pack or more of cigarettes per day?
9. Do you use chewing tobacco?
10. Do you drink pop daily (add an additional 2 points if you consume more than 3 cans daily)?
11. Do you take diuretics on a daily or weekly basis?
12. Do you take aspirin on a daily or weekly basis?
13. Do you take Tagamet or Zantac on a daily or weekly basis?
14. Do you use antacids on a daily basis?
15. Do you regularly use laxatives?
16. Do you take tetracycline on a daily or weekly basis?

17. Do you have a family history of heart disease, and/or have you been diagnosed with coronary artery/heart disease?
18. Do you have high blood pressure (above 140/90)?
19. Do you suffer from chronic diarrhea, Crohn's disease, and/or ulcerative colitis?
20. Do you have restless leg syndrome and/or nighttime leg cramps?
21. Do you snore excessively, and/or do you experience sleep apnea?
22. Do you suffer from angina attacks?
23. Do you take one or more heart medicines besides diuretics on a daily basis?
24. Do you have a history of muscle tearing?
25. Do you work with heavy metals, i.e. cadmium, mercury, lead, etc.?
26. Do you have severe leg, foot, and/or toe cramps?
27. Have you had one or more heart attacks in the past decade?
28. Do you have overactive or underactive thyroid function?
29. Do you have kidney stones, or have you had them in the past?

Your Score _____

Any score above five indicates a high risk for developing severe magnesium deficiency. Individuals who score above ten are at an extremely high risk, and if such individuals have a family history of heart disease, it is critical to make lifestyle alterations immediately. Follow the same instructions as were listed for the previous magnesium test. A score above 18 is of great concern; the risk for sudden death from cardiac disease is astronomically high. Individuals who score above ten should see a physician and have blood tests for determining magnesium levels. Magnesium is an intracellular nutrient.

Therefore, the serum level generally provides an inaccurate picture of tissue stores. Thus, both serum and intracellular levels should be assayed. However, blood tests are not the complete answer. It is possible to develop significant magnesium deficiency, even though blood tests are normal. Thus, the clinical picture, that is the symptoms and patient history, must be used as the final determinant for assessing the need for magnesium supplementation.

Manganese

Manganese is one of the least studied and understood of all nutrients. Nonetheless, its role in human nutrition is highly significant, as demonstrated by the crippling disease, a form of joint degeneration, that results from experimentally— induced manganese deficiency. As with other trace elements, manganese's primary role is that it is an enzyme activator. Dozens of enzymes, each with its own unique function, are dependent upon this mineral for optimal activity. For instance, the enzymes involved in cholesterol synthesis are manganese dependent, as are those involved in the synthesis of cartilage and bone. Regarding the latter the mucopolysaccharides, substances necessary for the formation of strong connective tissues, cannot be produced in the event of manganese deficiency.

Perhaps the most thoroughly documented and characteristic result of mild manganese deficiency is a specific syndrome of the joints known as slipped tendon disease or perosis. This is the result of a lack of skeletal maturation, leading to a slipping of the tendons off the joint and causing the characteristic "clicking" noise. These abnormalities are usually reversed by supplementing the diet with chelated manganese and manganese-rich foods.

Manganese is poorly absorbed from dietary sources. As much as 98% of ingested manganese is lost in the feces. Supplemental sources often fail to correct this, although chelated manganese products offer the best potential for absorption.

MANGANESE TEST

Which of these apply to you (each response worth 1 point)?

---

1. creaking and/or clicking of the joints
2. bone pain
3. arthritis and/or joint pain
4. infertility
5. thinning of the bones
6. brittle bones
7. increased susceptibility to infections
8. chronic knee, hip, and/or ankle pain
9. joints, which are easily injured
10. Are you a vegetarian? (If you are a vegan, add an additional 2 points)
11. Do you consume large amounts of bran, particularly wheat bran?
12. Do you have short stature (height under 5 feet) and/or growth impairment?
13. Are you a diabetic, and/or have you been diagnosed with an elevated blood sugar level?
14. Have you been diagnosed with hypoglycemia by blood testing (abnormal glucose tolerance test)?
15. Do you have a history of hepatitis and/or cirrhosis of the liver?
16. Do you consume sugar, pop, or candy on a daily or weekly basis?
17. Do you have low or high cholesterol?
18. Do you have a tendency to frequently sprain or injure your joints?
19. Do you have gout?
20. Are you obese?
21. Do you have a fracture or severe structural injury which has failed to heal?
22. Do you suffer from a blood-clotting abnormality?

23. Have you had a portion of your small intestine removed?
24. Do you have low levels of blood proteins, i.e. reduced globulin or albumin?
25. Do you eat mostly whole grains?

_____

Your Score _____

_____

1 to 4 points *Mild manganese deficiency*: Take 2 mg of chelated manganese and/or a multiple-vitamin/mineral containing manganese on a daily basis.

5 to 12 points *Moderate manganese deficiency*: Take 3 mg of chelated manganese morning and night and increase the consumption of manganese-rich foods. Avoid consuming the brans of grains; they contain phytates, which bind to manganese and prevent its absorption. Rice polishings and bran are a top source of this mineral. Take 3 heaping tablespoons of a rice polishings/bran drink mix, that is Nutri-Sense, daily.

13 and above *Severe manganese deficiency*: Take 3 mg of manganese three times daily (a total of 9 mg). To help enhance absorption take 2 tablespoons of lemon juice with each dosage. Increase the consumption of manganese-rich foods such as legumes, fresh meats, spices, blueberries, ginger, brown rice, rice polishings, rice bran, and nuts. Avoid dietary sources of phytates (e.g. whole wheat, corn bran, and oat bran). Drink mineral water, and avoid mineral depleted water, i.e. reverse osmosis, distilled, and soft water. Rice polishings and bran are a top source of this mineral. Take the rice polishings/rice bran complex, that is Nutri-Sense, 2 heaping tablespoons twice daily. Add a cup of blueberries to the Nutri-Sense with yogurt and make a manganese-rich drink mix: drink three or more cups daily.

Phosphorus

Phosphorus is a sort of Dr. Jekyll and Mr. Hyde of the minerals. This is because it is required for survival, yet can deal death. For instance, the flame in incandescent bulbs is white phosphorus; the heart of a match is made from red phosphorus; and certain pesticides are made from organic phosphate. However, without phosphorus, cells fail to divide, hearts stop beating, and reproduction halts.

Comprising approximately 1% of body weight, phosphorus is one of the most abundant substances in the human body. In fact, by itself it accounts for nearly one-fourth of the body's total mineral content. Of this amount 80% is bound to the bones and is a component of teeth.

Phosphorus is closely related to calcium in human nutrition. Like calcium, it requires vitamin D for absorption. A deficiency or an excess of phosphorus can upset calcium balance. Normally, the proportion of calcium to phosphorus in the bone is 2:1. However, the ratio within the soft tissues is a single molecule of calcium for every 20 molecules of phosphorus.

Dietary intake can play a major role in affecting tissue concentration of phosphate. Yet, few nutritional manuals emphasize the dietary need for phosphorus. Ensminger, et al., authors of *Food and Nutrition Encyclopedia,* aptly describe the crucial nature of phosphorus within the human body, stating: "Among the minerals essential to life, *none plays a more central role... It is found. . . in every cell; and it is involved in almost all, if not all, metabolic reactions* (italics mine)." Ensminger lists the functions of phosphorus as follows:

- It is required for bone formation and regeneration
- It is important in the development of teeth
- It is essential for normal milk secretion
- It is important for building muscle tissue
- It is involved in the synthesis of the genetic materials (RNA & DNA)

- It helps maintain acid-base and osmotic balance in the blood and within the cells
- It is essential for amino acid/protein metabolism
- It aids in the transport of fatty acids within the tissues
- It is crucial for the production of energy within the cells and muscles, including the heart
- It is an activator of many human enzyme systems

The proper utilization of phosphorus is dependent upon several factors. It should ideally be consumed in foods, like milk products, in a 2:1 ratio of calcium to phosphorous. It should also be present in a bio-available form. For instance, the phosphorus found in milk products and eggs is highly absorbable, while that found in whole grains is poorly absorbed. Whole grains contain fibrous compounds called phytates, which bind phosphates irreversibly. Thirdly, sufficient vitamin D must be available to ensure adequate calcium and phosphorus absorption from the gut. In fact, when sufficient vitamin D is available, the ratio of calcium to phosphorus becomes less crucial.

Phosphorus is found in a wide range of foods. Top sources include cheese, wheat germ, peanut flour, pumpkin and squash seeds, rice bran, rice polishings, soybean flour, organic liver, almonds, pistachios, sunflower seeds, and (organic) whole milk products.

PHOSPHORUS TEST

Which of these apply to you? (each response worth 1 point)

1. lack of appetite
2. anxiety
3. bone pain
4. loose teeth
5. teeth which crack and/or chip
6. irritability
7. numbness of the extremities

8. tremors
9. extreme fatigue
10. muscular weakness
11. swollen joints
12. chronic toothaches
13. gum disease (pyorrhea)
14. sluggish mental function
15. Do you consume refined sugar on a daily basis?
16. Do you avoid eating fresh vegetables, nuts, and seeds?
17. Do you have a history of infertility or low sperm count?
18. Do you have a history of coronary artery and/or heart disease?
19. Do you have osteoporosis?
20. Do you have more than four cavities?
21. Do you suffer from chronic joint pain (arthritis)?
22. Do you take antacids on a regular basis?
23. Do you have a duodenal ulcer, or have you had your duodenum removed?
24. Do you take cortisone orally on a regular basis?
25. Do you take iron pills on a daily basis?
26. Do you have chronic kidney problems?
27. Is your serum calcium low?
28. Do you have a history of a slipped or ruptured disk?
29. Do you follow a vegetarian diet devoid of milk products?
30. Do you have a problem building muscle tissue?
31. Have you experienced pica (desire to eat soil, clay, hair)?

Your Score _____

---

1 to 5 points *Mild Phosphorus deficiency*: A lack of phosphorus impairs energy production within every cell and organ of the body. The phosphorus deficiency can usually be corrected by increasing the intake of foods rich in this nutrient such as whole grains, almonds, pumpkin seeds, squash seeds, rice polishings, filberts, egg yolks, lean meats, rice bran, rice polishings, and fresh fish.

6 to 11 points *Moderate phosphorus deficiency*: In addition to the aforementioned take a multiple vitamin-mineral tablet containing phosphorus as well as vitamin D. Increase the consumption of vitamin D-rich foods, since this nutrient controls the rate at which phosphorus is absorbed. Eat snacks rich in phosphorus such as pumpkin seeds, sunflower seeds, pistachios, rice bran cookies, and cheese. As a concentrated vegetable source of phosphorus take Nutri-Sense, three heaping tablespoons daily in juice or water.

12 and above *Severe phosphorus deficiency*: Severe phosphorus deficiency may be a clue to the existence of hormonal disturbances. The parathyroid gland, which is located behind the thyroid gland at the back of the throat, produces parathyroid hormone. This hormone exerts potent control over the metabolism as well as absorption of phosphorus. Thus, a deficiency of this hormone leads to a decline in blood phosphorus levels. The adrenal glands also modulate phosphorus metabolism. Thus, a persistently low blood phosphorus level, despite attempts at dietary correction, is a signal of the existence of significant hormonal insufficiencies.

To correct this deficiency follow the previously mentioned advice and take 1,000 mg of phosphorus each day. In addition, take 800 to 1200 I.U. of vitamin D on a daily basis. Prolonged consumption of antacids induces phosphorus depletion which may be so severe that it is life-threatening. This syndrome is characterized by weakness, loss of appetite, and bone pain. Avoid antacids, cortisone, alcohol, refined sugar, and iron supplements, all of which impede phosphorus absorption. It may be necessary to monitor phosphorus status via blood testing. If the phosphorus level fails to normalize, medical evaluation for hormonal deficiencies may be necessary. As a concentrated vegetable source of phosphorus take Nutri-Sense, four heaping tablespoons daily in juice or water.

Potassium

No mineral can be deemed more crucial for survival than potassium. Without it, death rapidly results from sudden cardiac arrest. Potassium is the heart's nerve firing agent, initiating impulses to stimulate contraction of the heart muscle fibers. Therefore, the heart is dependent upon this mineral in order to pump in its unending fashion. Moreover, potassium helps control the function of every nerve in the body. Thus, a deficiency of this mineral would have a negative impact upon the function of every organ, in fact, every cell in the body.

Fresh tree-ripened fruits and vegetables are rich in potassium, but the top sources on a per weight basis are spices, particularly coriander, cumin, basil, parsley, ginger, hot pepper, dill weed, tarragon, paprika, and turmeric. Nuts, seeds, and legumes are also rich sources.

Potassium deficiency is a proven contributing cause of a number of illnesses, including:

arthritis	irritable bowel syndrome
kidney stones	Alzheimer's disease
atrial fibrillation	multiple sclerosis
celiac disease	myasthenia gravis
bundle branch block	Crohn's disease
high blood pressure	lupus
coronary artery disease	atherosclerosis
ulcerative colitis	diabetes
hypothyroidism	stroke
adrenal insufficiency	

Individuals who are taking high blood pressure medications are most vulnerable to developing potassium deficiency, since these agents cause the spillage of large quantities of this mineral into the urine. Physicians often attempt to minimize this by prescribing potassium-sparing diuretics. However, the most commonly prescribed diuretics aggressively deplete tissue stores of potassium, causing a drug-induced systemic potassium deficiency.

The thiazide diuretics, a category which includes Diazide and chlorothiazide, cause the loss of untold millions of molecules of potassium for every pill taken. This is one reason that diuretic usage is associated with sudden death syndrome. The fact is certain studies, including the MRFIT trial reported in the journal *Science* (October 1982), warn of the dangers of long-term diuretic usage. Such studies document how individuals who fail to take diuretics for high blood pressure live significantly longer than hypertensive patients who take medications.

POTASSIUM TEST

Which of these apply to you (each response worth 1 point)?

1. acne
2. arthritis and/or swollen joints
3. constipation
4. impaired intellect
5. depression
6. memory loss
7. edema (swelling) of the extremities
8. agitation and/or irritability
9. low blood pressure
10. irregular heartbeat
11. rapid heartbeat
12. frequent urination with large volumes
13. blood sugar disturbances
14. constant fatigue
15. muscular weakness
16. nervousness
17. muscle cramps
18. lightheadedness and/or episodes of fainting
19. twitching of the muscles and/or tremors
20. intolerance to exercise and/or lack of a desire to exercise
21. poor appetite

22. chronic headaches
23. sudden episodes of paralysis
24. Do you consume alcohol on a daily basis (add an additional 2 points)?
25. Do you consume fresh fruits, vegetables, nuts, and seeds only occasionally?
26. Do you take antacids or Zantac/Tagamet on a daily basis?
27. Do you use diuretics on a daily or weekly basis?
28. Do you have high blood pressure (greater than 140/90)?
29. Have you had a stroke, or do you suffer from TIAs (transient ischemic attacks)?
30. Do you have a history of angina, heart disease, and/or hardening of the arteries?
31. Do you consume aspirin, Motrin, or similar anti-inflammatory drugs on a daily or weekly basis?
32. Do you take commercial laxatives daily or weekly (add an additional 2 points)?
33. Do you suffer from chronic or intermittent diarrhea?
34. Are you currently taking drugs containing cortisone?
35. Do you consume refined sugars on a daily basis (add an additional 2 points)?
36. Do you experience abdominal bloating?
37. Do you have swelling of the eyelids or swelling under the eyes?
38. Do you vomit frequently (once a week or more)?
39. Are you a diabetic?

Your Score _____

---

1 to 8 points *Mild potassium deficiency*: Enrich the diet with top food sources of potassium. Excellent food sources include dried fruit, bananas, cantaloupe, tomato juice, and broccoli. In addition, take a multiple-mineral tablet containing potassium. Try the Potassium Shake in the recipe section.

9 to 19 points *Moderate potassium deficiency*: In addition to the previously mentioned advice, take a daily dosage of 1 or 2 tablets of potassium gluconate twice daily. Eat a cup of organic raisins or dried apricots daily. Eat also a banana daily.

20 and above *Severe potassium deficiency*: Warning—severe potassium deficit may lead to cardiac rhythm disturbances. If the blood potassium level drops excessively low, sudden cardiac standstill may result. Before beginning supplementation have your blood potassium level assessed. If blood levels are normal or slightly depressed, take 2 or 3 potassium gluconate tablets twice daily. In the event of severe potassium deficiency medical intervention is necessary. Proper care might include potassium medication plus frequent monitoring of the blood potassium level. However, there is a word of caution: potassium drugs, especially tablets, may be caustic and can cause ulcerations of the intestines. To avoid this opt for liquid forms of potassium or utilize less toxic forms such as the non-prescription potassium gluconate. Eat potassium-rich foods every day. Consume one or more cups of organic raisins or dried apricots daily. Prepare large batches of the potassium-rich fruit and/or vegetable salads and eat the salads daily. If you develop symptoms of heart rhythm disturbances, such as skipped beats, slow heart rate, rapid heart rate or chest pains, see your doctor immediately.

Selenium

As important as potassium is for saving lives from sudden death, so is selenium indispensable for preventing deaths of a different kind: those due to chronic degenerative diseases. Selenium is one of Nature's most important cancer-blocking agents. Studies have shown that cancer is far less prevalent in regions with high water and soil content of selenium than in regions where selenium is not found. In addition, cancer patients have lower blood and tissue levels of selenium than healthy individuals.

Selenium also offers significant protection against heart disease. Recent studies document that individuals with low tissue levels of selenium are at a higher risk for heart attacks than those whose selenium levels are normal.

The protective effects of selenium are due largely to its potent antioxidant function. Antioxidants prevent the tissue damage which occurs as a result of oxidation. Thus, selenium helps stall the aging process. What's more, it prevents the onset of diseases of civilization such as arthritis, diabetes, multiple sclerosis, lupus, heart disease, and cancer. In fact, researchers have discovered that this mineral not only blocks the oxidative processes that lead to these diseases but also may reverse the damage after it occurs.

Selenium offers protection against heavy metal toxicity. It helps the body eliminate heavy metals by increasing the rate of their excretion in the urine and feces. Selenium is a particularly effective antidote for chronic mercury intoxication.

Selenium is a powerful immune enhancing agent. It greatly accelerates the ability of white blood cells to destroy invaders. In addition, the production of the human body's crucial anti-allergy and anti-microbial proteins, the antibodies, are significantly enhanced as a result of selenium therapy.

This mineral's ability to strengthen immunity may be the explanation behind its anti-allergy action. Virtually all chronic allergy patients improve after increasing the intake of selenium, regardless of the type of allergies from which they suffer.

Individuals who are chronically exposed to radiation require elevated dosages of selenium. Unfortunately, hundreds of thousands of Americans are being exposed to chronic radioactivity. A listing of such individuals includes x-ray technicians, nuclear power plant employees, uranium miners, nuclear waste disposal workers, individuals undergoing routine x-rays, dentists and dental technicians, radiologists, surgeons, chiropractors and chiropractic technicians, interns/residents, radiological nurses, food irradiation plant workers, clock and watch laborers who work with radium, podiatrists, video game enthusiasts, and computer operators.

Now that mail is being irradiated postal workers are developing a wide arrange of radiation-induced illnesses. So are corporate mail handlers. Apparently, terrorism was used as a ruse to sell multi-million dollar irradiation equipment. Additionally, individuals living within a thirty mile radius of a nuclear plant are subjected to excessive radiation exposure.[9] Certainly, all such individuals should supplement their diets with selenium.

The selenium content of food depends entirely upon soil levels. Thus, it is difficult to produce a comprehensive listing of selenium-rich foods. However, the finest sources are fresh meats, vegetables, nuts, seeds, and mushrooms. For instance, the selenium content of beef raised in South Dakota, a region rich in selenium, may be several times greater than beef raised in Indiana, a region where the soil is devoid of selenium.

It is truly the dilemma of modern man that food is only as healthy and nutrient-rich as the soil upon which it is grown. As little as two hundred years ago virtually all of the soil in the world could have been regarded as virgin. However, commercial farming, with its emphasis on synthetic agrichemicals, has devastated the health of the soil. Thus, while certain vegetables, such as garlic, radishes, and turnips, are traditionally regarded as rich sources of selenium, this would hold true only if the vegetables were grown in selenium-rich soil. Furthermore, even if the soil is rich in selenium, commercial fertilizers and chemical treatments may prevent the absorption of selenium into plants.

Nearly one third of the states have selenium-deficient soil. Many of these states have such a high cancer incidence that they are known collectively as the cancer belt. This region includes primarily the states surrounding the Great Lakes: Wisconsin, Illinois, Indiana, Ohio, Michigan, and Western New York. Also

---

9. The heightened risk for cancer in those exposed to radiation from nuclear power plants is no longer an uncertainty. For instance, a recent study published in England documented a tenfold increase in leukemia in children fathered by nuclear power plant employees.

included in the cancer belt are the Canadian provinces of Manitoba, Ontario, and Quebec; the latter two border the northern edges of the Great Lakes. Additionally, numerous coastal states, such as Washington, Oregon, Maine, Massachusetts, Connecticut, Rhode Island, Vermont, New Jersey, the Carolinas, West Virginia, and Florida, have selenium-deficient soil. Individuals living in these regions should routinely supplement their diets with an organically bound form of selenium (e.g. selenium-kelp, seleno-methionine, or selenium-yeast).

SELENIUM TEST

Which of these apply to you (each response worth 1 point)?

1. tendency to be allergic to foods, drugs, or chemicals
2. premature aging
3. loss of skin elasticity (excessive wrinkling)
4. raised brownish lesions on the face, back, abdomen, or legs
5. infertility or low sperm count
6. increased susceptibility to yeast/fungal infections
7. acne
8. increased susceptibility to colds, flu, or other infections
9. hair loss
10. prostate problems
11. delayed wound healing
12. dermatitis and/or eczema
13. chronic urinary tract infections
14. Do you consume alcoholic beverages on a daily basis?
15. Do you live in a large city affected by heavy smog?
16. Are you developing an increasing number of moles and/or liver spots?
17. Do you suffer from cataracts and/or macular degeneration?
18. Do you have a history of asthma, hives, throat swelling, or other severe allergic reactions?

19. Do you have a history of coronary artery disease, cardiomyopathy (i.e. heart muscle degeneration), atherosclerosis, and/or high blood pressure?
20. Do you have arthritis affecting several joints?
21. Do you suffer from inhalant allergies such as hay fever, toxic, and mold sensitivity?
22. Are you highly sensitive to chemical smells, like perfumes, gas fumes, etc?
23. Do you have silver fillings in your teeth?
24. Do you have a history of internal and/or external cancer?
25. Do you suffer from chronic fungal infections?
26. Do you have hepatitis?
27. Do you suffer from insulin-dependent diabetes?
28. Do you live in one of the low-selenium states located in the cancer belt?
29. Are you exposed to heavy concentrations of toxic chemicals or heavy metals (mercury, silver, lead, etc.)?
30. Do you have pancreatitis?
31. Are you a mail-sorter or postal worker, who handles large quantities of mail?

Your Score _____

---

1 to 6 points *Mild selenium deficiency*: Selenium deficiency, even in a mild state, must be regarded seriously. One reason is that selenium protects the human body from toxic chemical exposure, heavy metal overload, radiation, and excessive sunlight. However, equally important is the fact that even a modest decline in selenium levels results in a corresponding decline in immune function.

Organically bound selenium is the ideal supplemental source. In fact, it is the only type which can be consumed in the doses suggested herein. Avoid sodium selenite; it is toxic, even in relatively small dosages. On a daily basis take 200 mcg of organically bound selenium. Vitamin E potentiates the action of selenium. Therefore, also take 400 I. U. of natural source vitamin E. Or, to get vitamin E in a natural unprocessed form take two to four tablespoons Pumpkinol daily (vitamin E now is derived from genetically engineered soy, which may cause toxicity). Increase consumption of selenium-rich foods, particularly radishes, turnips, carrots, raw nuts, and seeds.

7 to 14 points *Moderate selenium deficiency*: Follow the previously mentioned advice, and increase the dosage of selenium to 400 mcg daily. Reduce this dosage to 300 mcg daily after one month. In addition, increase the intake of vitamin E to a minimum of 800 I.U. daily, as the extra vitamin E will help conserve selenium, preventing its destruction by noxious agents. Or, as a natural source, take Pumpkinol, four to six tablespoons daily.

15 and above *Severe selenium deficiency*: Warning— prolonged selenium deficit increases the risks for a variety of serious diseases, particularly cancer, heart disease, and arthritis. Immune impairment and allergic diseases are also associated with selenium deficiency. Take 500 mcg of organically bound selenium each day. Curtail the consumption of alcoholic beverages and eliminate refined sugar, flour, and rice from the diet. Increase the intake of raw vegetables, nuts, seeds, and whole grains, particularly brown rice. Take 1200 I.U. of vitamin E (or six tablespoons Pumpkinol) and 2,000 mg of vitamin C daily. After one month reduce the dosage of selenium to 400 mcg per day. After 90 days take a maintenance level of 200 mcg daily. Do not take megadoses of inorganic selenium, since it may cause toxicity.

Silicon

More abundant in the body than iron or calcium, silicon has recently been decreed essential to human nutrition. It is essential for the development of all connective tissues, including the tendons, ligaments, arterial walls, skin, and bones. Furthermore, it assists in maintaining bone hardness as well as flexibility. In fact, joint damage, degeneration, and/or deformity are primary symptoms of silicon deficiency.

Silicon is the most abundant mineral found in the earth's crust. However, despite its abundance in soil and water, the deficiency is common in America. That is because this mineral is found in large quantities only in pure unprocessed foods and fresh unpolluted water. How many Americans have a diet rich in these?

Perhaps the most celebrated role of this mineral in human nutrition relates to its importance in the maintenance of healthy connective tissues: skin, hair, nails, joints, and bones. This is one reason there is a surging interest within the cosmetic industry for lotions, creams, and shampoos containing silicon (in the form of silica) as a primary active ingredient. Top dietary sources of silicon include well water, bottled mineral water, garden-fresh vegetables, fresh milk products, fresh whole grains, organic liver, and fresh lean meats. Additionally, wild game and wild herbs are exceptionally rich in silicon.

SILICON TEST

Which of these apply to you (each response worth 1 point)?

1. brittle hair, split ends, and/or nails
2. hair loss
3. thin hair
4. impaired wound healing
5. varicose veins
6. high blood pressure
7. dry flaky skin
8. brittle bones and/or osteoporosis
9. dermatitis, psoriasis, and/or eczema

10. skin which breaks open easily
11. chronic lower back pain
12. weak joints and/or ligaments
13. rapidly aging skin
14. loss of skin elasticity
15. joint swelling and/or deformity
16. poor circulation
17. eczema
18. Do you drink softened water on a regular basis?
19. Do you consume refined sugar on a daily basis?
20. Do you have a history of heart or circulatory disease?
21. Do you drink reverse osmosis or distilled water on a regular basis?
22. Do you have a history of a collagen disease such as scleroderma, rheumatoid arthritis, fibromyositis, or lupus?
23. Are you a diabetic?
24. Do you have chronic lung infections?
25. Do you suffer from premature graying of the hair?
26. Do you have osteoporosis (thinning of the bones)?

Your Score _____

---

1 to 6 points *Mild silicon deficiency*: Take 1,000 mg of organic silica daily. Avoid refined sugars. Drink mineral, tap (purified), or well water; distilled, softened, and reverse osmosis water are devoid of silicon.

7 to 14 points *Moderate silicon deficiency*: Take 2,000 mg of organic silica daily. Avoid distilled, reverse osmosis, or softened water and drink mineral water instead. Curtail the consumption of refined sugar and flour; increase the consumption of raw and/or unprocessed foods.

15 and above *Severe silicon deficiency*: A systemic deficiency of silicon increases the risks for heart disease, arthritis, osteoporosis, balding, eczema, psoriasis, and cancer. Take 3,000 mg of organic silica daily and follow the recommendations suggested for mild-moderate deficiencies. Curtail the consumption of refined sugars, alcoholic beverages, white flour, and other processed foods. Eat wild game as often as possible, and consume several helpings each day of raw vegetables, nuts, and/or seeds.

Sodium

Much has been written in nutritional/medical circles about sodium, but it has largely been negative. This is unfortunate, since this mineral is essential to human existence. Though it may be a surprise to many people, sodium is a necessary nutrient for the preservation of optimal health. Historians note that many centuries ago salt was so valuable that men traded it for its weight in gold. In contrast, the medical profession teaches that salt is dangerous and that the public should avoid it at all costs. While it is true that certain individuals are salt-sensitive and must curb their intake, the majority of Americans would suffer no ill effects by keeping salt in their diets.

The frequent prescription of the low sodium diet may, in fact, be dangerous. Sodium deficiency is surprisingly common in Americans. In certain individuals the deficiency becomes so extreme that blood levels dip below the normal range. This is a consequence of a condition known as the *Sodium Wasting Syndrome*. I discovered this syndrome in 1987 in Arlington Heights, Illinois, while treating patients in my clinic. Individuals with this condition lose sodium into the urine in large amounts and, despite an excess of sodium in the diet, ultimately become sodium deficient. They literally lose sodium as fast as they consume it. Such individuals are particularly vulnerable to the development of the deficiency when placed on sodium-restricted diets. They may become so grossly deficient in this mineral that they develop a variety of symptoms seemingly so vague that doctors usually brush them off as "psychological". Yet, these patients are ill as a result of a lack of sodium, since this mineral is essential for maintaining such critical functions as the blood electrolyte balance, cardiac tone and pumping power, nerve firing, and digestive juice synthesis.

Sodium wasting is a significant health malady. This mineral exerts numerous critical functions within human tissues, and low blood levels of sodium must not be regarded lightly. For instance, when sodium is wasted, there is also a decrease in tissue fluid. The latter phenomenon is known as volume depletion and is defined as a massive loss of fluid and electrolytes from the blood and cells. In other words, sodium is an anti-dehydrating agent.

Volume depletion is largely what happens in heat exhaustion and heat stroke. In this potentially fatal circumstance the loss of water as well as electrolytes, such as sodium bicarbonate, magnesium, and potassium, occurs. Ideally, treatment should include water and electrolyte replacement. In fact, drinking an excess of mineral-depleted water may precipitate heat exhaustion by a "washing out" effect, leading to a reduction in serum electrolyte levels. Thus, in the case of the sodium waster, dietary salt is necessary to help maintain fluid balance and prevent excessive loss of water from the tissues.

Low levels of sodium can be confirmed by blood testing. The fact is when blood levels are persistently low, it may be necessary to prescribe sodium as a therapeutic agent. I have frequently recommended that patients who suffer from the Sodium Wasting Syndrome use a heavy hand with the salt shaker (a good sea salt) and certainly should salt their food to taste, without concern.

The majority of individuals with the Sodium Wasting Syndrome have developed it as a consequence of suffering from a chronic debilitating condition known as *adrenal insufficiency.* The adrenal glands produce the body's sodium preserver, a hormone called *aldosterone.* This hormone "instructs" the kidneys to retain sodium by keeping it in the bloodstream and preventing it from being lost into the urine. Without adequate amounts of aldosterone, untold millions of molecules of sodium are spilled into the urine every minute. Salt is needed to maintain the strength of the circulatory system. Thus, it must be continually replenished via the diet, although an additional approach would be to take aldosterone, a prescription drug.

However, the key to normalizing the sodium level is to enhance adrenal function through improved diet and nutritional supplementation. With improved adrenal function sodium wasting is reduced or may be halted entirely.

Sea salt is preferable over table salt for several reasons. Table salt contains additives, including sugar (as dextrose) and aluminum. The aluminum prevents caking, and the sugar is probably added to make the taste of salt more appealing. In addition to being additive-free, sea salt contains a plethora of minerals besides sodium. Both sea salt and iodized table salt are rich sources of iodine. A very real concern is that sea salt may contain residues of toxic chemicals. To minimize this purchase sea salt which is collected from regions other than the coastal United States. One of the best sources of sea salt is *Celtic Salt* from France. It is the least processed of all sea salts and retains an exceptionally high and diversified mineral content. Another option is land-derived salts. One of the finest is *Real Salt,* a pollutant-free salt extracted from an ancient seabed in Utah. Check your local health food store for these salts. However, Real Salt must be supplemented with other salt sources. This is because the former, being ancient, has lost all its iodine.

SODIUM TEST

Which of these apply to you (each response worth 1 point)?

1. confusion and/or hallucinations
2. seizures
3. muscular weakness
4. lethargy and/or fatigue
5. lack of appetite
6. muscle cramps
7. headaches
8. excessive urination and/or urge to urinate from stress
9. cold weather causes urge to urinate
10. diarrhea
11. cold extremities
12. paranoia
13. psychotic behavior
14. low blood pressure
15. nausea and/or vomiting
16. dizziness
17. apathy
18. lack of thirst
19. lips dry and cracking
20. Is your blood cholesterol level low?
21. Do you have a tendency to become dehydrated?
22. Do you adhere to a sodium-restricted diet?
23. Do you take diuretics on a daily or weekly basis?
24. Do you drink distilled and/or reverse osmosis water on a regular basis?
25. Do you crave salt or salty foods?
26. Have you been diagnosed with Addison's disease and/or adrenal insufficiency?
27. Do you exercise vigorously several times per week?
28. Are you unusually sensitive to heat, especially hot, humid weather, saunas, hot tubs, etc.?
29. Do you have difficulty digesting meat and other protein-rich foods?

30. Is your serum sodium low (below 139 mg/dl)?
31. Do you suffer from lack of concentration or memory loss?

Your Score _____

1 to 5 points *Mild sodium deficiency*: All that usually needs to be done at this stage is to increase the consumption of salt and salty foods. Take also pantothenic acid, 500 mg daily.

6 to 11 points *Moderate sodium deficiency*: Individuals who score in this category and who adhere to a low sodium diet should add sodium to their diets and use a heavy hand with the salt shaker. Take 1,000 mg of pantothenic acid daily, since this helps stimulate the synthesis of aldosterone, the adrenal hormone which helps conserve sodium. Also, as a natural vitamin C source take Flavin-C, 4 caps daily. Natural vitamin C is needed for adrenal gland regeneration. Be sure to eat salty snacks between meals and use salt in all cooking. Also, to help the body conserve salt it is crucial to strengthen adrenal function. As a high grade royal jelly supplement take Royal Kick, 4 caps every morning.

12 to 20 points *Severe sodium deficiency*: Fill 2 gelatin capsules with sea salt and take the salt capsules with every meal. Salt all foods to taste. Take 1,000 to 2,000 mg of pantothenic acid and 1,000 mg of vitamin C (i.e. Flavin-C) each day. (Note: only natural vitamin C helps regenerate the adrenal glands) In addition, be sure to consume plenty of foods rich in cholesterol; aldosterone is made from cholesterol. Also, to help the body conserve salt it is crucial to strengthen adrenal function. As a high grade royal jelly source take Royal Kick, 6 caps every morning.

21 and above *Extreme sodium deficiency*: Follow the previously mentioned recommendations. Fill 3 to 4 gelatin capsules with sea salt and liberally salt all foods. Eat salty snacks between meals such as salted roasted nuts, sunflower seeds, olives, and pickles. Be sure to eliminate all dietary sources of refined sugar, since sugar places stress upon the adrenal glands leading to a depletion of aldosterone stores. Also, to help the body conserve salt it is crucial to strengthen adrenal function. As a source of high grade royal jelly take Royal Kick, 4 caps twice daily. Also, take pantothenic acid capsules, 300 mg twice daily in divided doses. Take a natural vitamin C supplement, that is Flavin-C, three or more caps twice daily.

Note: The symptoms of sodium deficiency are subtle. Therefore, it is possible to develop a number of these symptoms, even though blood tests are normal. Often, doctors miss the diagnosis. What's more, certain individuals may be sensitive to sodium, particularly those suffering from hypertension, kidney disease, or fluid retention. Such individuals should not add large amounts of sodium to their diets. They may instead try small amounts of sea salt to tolerance. If you have a history of any of these diseases or if you are wary of consuming sodium, get a blood chemistry panel which includes a serum sodium level. If the level is normal or high-normal, use only moderate amounts of salt. If the level is below 140 (as milliliters per deciliter), sodium-wasting is likely. Levels below 138 confirm the diagnosis of the Sodium Wasting Syndrome.

Sodium levels often improve or normalize as a result of nutritional therapy. Thus, the need for salt replacement may diminish. If your sodium level is low, have the level rechecked approximately 60 days after beginning this program. When the level normalizes, stop consuming supplemental salt; instead, use salt to taste. To strengthen the adrenal glands take Royal Kick, six caps every morning.

Zinc

Zinc is one of the most heavily researched of all nutrients. It is perhaps most renowned for its role in immunity; even mild zinc deficiency leads to impairment of the immune response. For men zinc is known particularly as the anti-prostatitis nutrient. Stress causes a rapid depletion of tissue zinc levels. Wounds and injuries fail to heal normally in the event of zinc deficiency. This is true of a wide range of injuries, including cuts, bruises, abrasions, bed sores, ulcers (internal and external), sprains, and fractures.

Surgical patients are vulnerable for developing zinc deficiency, and the post-surgical period is the worst time for this to occur. Such patients desperately need zinc for healing and for preventing post-surgical infections. A few surgeons have recognized this dilemma and are infusing zinc along with other critical nutrients by vein after surgery.

Not only do wounds heal slowly when zinc is deficient, but they are also highly likely to become infected. In zinc-deficient children minor cuts could result in pus-filled wounds or even sepsis (blood poisoning). Additionally, impetigo and various other staph infections, as well as acne, are correlated with poor zinc nutriture. Adults may suffer similar consequences. Individuals who repeatedly develop boils, infected cysts, fingernail bed infections (paronychia), and staph/strep infections are invariably zinc deficient. Further, individuals who suffer from repeated bouts of the flu, pneumonia, ear infections, tonsillitis, or sore throats, or who fail to recover rapidly after such infections, are in all likelihood severely deficient in this mineral.

Molecularly, zinc is a rather large mineral. Less than 30% of the zinc ingested via food is absorbed into the blood. Absorption from zinc supplements may be as low as 5 to 10%.

The duodenum is the primary site of absorption. Absorption declines significantly in those suffering from digestive diseases, particularly diseases affecting the upper portion of the small intestine. Thus, in individuals afflicted with duodenal ulcer, intestinal worms, giardia infection, grain allergies (gluten intolerance), and Crohn's disease, absorption is often minimal, and extreme zinc deficiency usually occurs.

Certain drugs, notably alcohol, diuretics, cortisone, Tagamet, Zantac, and antacids, significantly impair zinc absorption. Ensminger states that alcohol may "precipitate a zinc deficiency by flushing...zinc out of the liver and into the urine."

Certain foods impair zinc absorption. Whole grains contain the zinc antagonist called phytic acid (pl. *phytates*). Beans and lentils contain certain fibrous compounds, which destroy zinc. Because of the large concentration of phytates, plant protein, when ingested in large amounts, is one of the most common causes of zinc deficit. In particular, soy protein aggressively induces zinc deficiency. Soybeans are unusually rich in copper, which is a zinc antagonist. Thus, vegetarians who eat primarily soy as a protein source frequently develop zinc deficiency.

Zinc is a crucial component of a wide range of human enzyme systems. Without it, the enzymes are rendered inoperable. Zinc-dependent enzymes control the following functions:

a) digestion of protein
b) fatty acid metabolism
c) sugar metabolism
d) bone deposition
e) skin cell formation synthesis
f) hair growth
g) sex hormone synthesis
h) insulin synthesis
i) thymic hormone synthesis

When food is processed, zinc is rapidly destroyed. Thus, only wholesome unprocessed food can be relied upon to provide adequate amounts. As much as 80% of the zinc is lost when whole grains are refined. Similar losses result when fruits and vegetables are canned or frozen. However, organically grown produce and grains contain up to ten times the zinc of commercially grown food. Top sources of zinc include crab, herring, liver, lobster, oysters, lamb, turkey, poppy seeds, caraway seeds, and whole grains.

ZINC TEST

Which of these apply to you (each response worth 1 point)?

1. lack of appetite or anorexia
2. lack of taste
3. white spots on the fingernails (add an additional 2 points if the spots are excessive)
4. reduced sperm count and/or infertility
5. lack of the sense of smell
6. chronic or recurrent ear infections
7. acne
8. slow growing hair and/or nails
9. increased susceptibility to colds, flu, or other infections
10. hair loss
11. prostate problems (prostatitis)
12. delayed wound healing
13. geographic tongue
14. growth impairment (stunted growth)
15. light-colored pigment in the hair
16. dermatitis
17. blood sugar disturbances
18. dry and/or brittle hair
19. excessively dry or oily skin
20. sties on the eyelids
21. stretch marks
22. premature graying of the hair
23. irregular menstrual cycles (especially in teenagers)
24. impotence (lack of erection)
25. delayed sexual maturity
26. growing pains (or aching joints in teenagers)
27. sore or inflamed cracks in the skin at the fingertips
28. hangnails
29. chapped or split lips
30. recurrent vaginal yeast infections
31. sensitivity of the eyes to light

32. enlarged facial pores
33. Do you consume refined sugars on a daily basis?
34. Do you consume alcoholic beverages on a daily or weekly basis?
35. Are you a diabetic?
36. Do you develop canker sores or other oral ulcerations?
37. Do you have a history of gout?
38. Do you consume large amounts of whole grains and/or grain brans on a daily basis?
39. Do you take diuretics on a daily or weekly basis?
40. Do you suffer from repeated bouts of chronic skin infections?
41. Do you suffer from recurrent urinary tract infections?
42. Does your skin sunburn easily, or do you develop sun-induced rashes?
43. Do you have difficulty digesting meat or other protein-rich foods?
44. Do you have a history of detached retina or retinal bleeding?
45. Do you have macular degeneration?
46. Do you exercise vigorously on a daily basis?
47. Have you experienced prolonged periods of psychic stress?
48. Do you develop urinary tract infections frequently?
49. Do you suffer from duodenal ulcer, or have you had your duodenum removed?
50. Do you suffer from pancreatic disease?
51. Do you suffer from osteoporosis?
52. Do you have biliary sclerosis and/or hepatitis?
53. Do you take cortisone on a daily or weekly basis?
54. Do you take birth control pills?
55. Do you take large amounts of supplemental calcium on a daily basis?

Your Score _____

---

1 to 7 points *Mild zinc deficiency*: Take a multiple vitamin-mineral tablet containing zinc, and increase the consumption of zinc-rich foods.

8 to 16 points *Moderate zinc deficiency*: In addition to the multiple vitamin-mineral supplement take 30 mg of zinc daily. Consume zinc-rich foods on a daily basis. Avoid the brans of grains in order to reduce the consumption of phytates, which bind zinc and prevent its absorption. Particularly, avoid wheat bran. Curtail the consumption of all dietary sources of refined sugars, and, if you drink alcohol regularly, quit.

17 to 29 points *Severe zinc deficiency*: Follow the aforementioned advice. Zinc deficiency greatly impairs immune response. Individuals suffering from this level of deficiency are vulnerable to the development of a variety of infections, particularly yeast infections, urinary tract infections, tuberculosis, influenza, and the common cold. Follow the previously mentioned measures and take 75 mg of zinc daily. After two months reduce this dosage to 50 mg daily. Alcohol, refined flour, and refined sugar should be completely avoided. Also, avoid the intake of all soy products. At this dosage be sure to take supplemental copper (4 mg per day).

30 and above *Extreme zinc deficiency*: Warning—zinc is essential to the synthesis of genetic material and is, therefore, required for cellular growth. Furthermore, protein synthesis throughout all tissues is dependent upon this mineral. Thus, at this level of deficiency cellular damage will readily occur.

It is crucial to correct this zinc deficiency immediately. Moreover, further losses of zinc must be minimized. Follow the aforementioned advice. Avoid substances which deplete zinc, which include alcohol, refined sugar, white flour, white rice, coffee, sugar-sweetened soda pops, and certain drugs, notably diuretics and birth control pills. In the daily menus increase the consumption of foods rich in zinc. However, avoid consuming excessive amounts of whole grains and grain fibers, such as wheat, corn, or oat bran, since they bind zinc and may induce a deficiency by preventing its absorption. In addition to dietary sources, take 75 to 100 mg of zinc daily. Because this is megadose therapy, be sure to take 2 mg of copper morning and night. The copper is needed because when zinc is taken in large doses, copper absorption is severely impaired. Thus, a secondary copper deficiency may result from prolonged megadose zinc therapy. Alcohol and medicinal diuretics are especially dangerous, since they aggressively flush zinc into the urine.[10]

Para Amino Benzoic Acid (PABA)

Para amino benzoic acid is actually a derivative of folic acid. In fact, creams rich in PABA can be used to treat sunburn, since PABA is a powerful antioxidant for stimulating tissue healing. However, as a separate substance it has its own important actions. Research has found that PABA is exceptionally valuable for blocking the ill effects of sunlight on the skin. It has also been discovered that PABA has an anti-graying action for the hair and not only prevents premature graying but may also actually restore hair to its original color. What's more, it plays an important role in the prevention of hair loss. Because of these functions, it may be regarded as the "healthy hair and skin" vitamin. PABA is found in the same food sources as folic acid.

Certain individuals may be allergic to PABA. This allergy often manifests as an intolerance to sunscreens containing it. If you are one of these PABA-sensitive individuals, internal consumption is contraindicated. In this instance the health benefits of PABA may be achieved through the use of folic acid, since this vitamin is closely related to it and possesses many of its functions.

---

10. To determine a zinc deficiency is quite easy. There is a nutritional zinc test called Zinc Tally. It is a liquid form of zinc, and, depending on the taste or lack of taste, this indicates the level of zinc sufficiency or deficiency. Zinc Tally may be found in many health food stores.

PARA AMINO BENZOIC ACID (PABA) TEST

Which of these apply to you (each response worth 1 point)?

1. premature graying of the hair
2. vitiligo (tiny white spots on the skin due to loss of pigment)
3. depression
4. chronic fatigue
5. chronic headaches
6. nervousness and/or irritability
7. skin rashes and/or dermatitis
8. hair loss
9. constipation
10. Do you take sulfa drugs (for bacterial infections) on a monthly, weekly, or daily basis?
11. Do you regularly take antibiotics (besides sulfa drugs)?
12. Do you sunburn easily?
13. Do you suffer from irritable bowel syndrome, ulcerative colitis, Crohn's disease, and/or celiac disease?
14. Have you had a portion of your intestines removed?
15. Do you have a history of autoimmune disease, (thyroiditis, endometriosis, fibromyositis, polymyositis, diabetes, or lupus)?
16. Is your skin aging rapidly?
17. Do you suffer from an excessive amount of age or liver spots?
18. Are you constantly being exposed to radiation or x-rays?

Your Score _____

1 to 4 points *Mild PABA deficiency*: Take 200 mg of PABA daily and use sunscreens containing PABA.

5 to 10 points *Moderate PABA deficiency*: Whenever you are exposed to the sun be sure to use sunscreens containing PABA. Take 500 mg of PABA twice daily along with 2 mg of folic acid daily, since this helps conserve PABA. Take also a source of crude rice fractions, e.g. Nutri-Sense, one or two heaping tablespoons daily.

11 and above *Severe PABA deficiency*: Take 1,000 mg of PABA twice daily. If you are suffering from vitiligo, severe graying of the hair, and/or hair loss, increase the dosage to 3 grams (3000 mg) daily. If there is no response, try 5 grams of PABA and add 5 mg of folic acid. Whenever you are exposed to the sun, use sunscreens containing PABA. Again, there is a word of caution. Individuals who react to PABA in sunscreens may also be sensitive to oral consumption: If you are reactive, stop all oral doses of PABA. Take also a source of crude rice fractions, such as Nutri-Sense, two or three heaping tablespoons daily.

Amino Acids

Amino acids are a group of nutrients which are derived from proteins in our foods. They are a rather large group of compounds; over forty are known in Nature. This means that there is a greater number of amino acids than all the vitamins and minerals combined.

All proteins in the human body—enzymes, hair, skin, or the cells of the internal organs—consist of amino acids. They are truly the functional and structural building blocks of the human system. Thus, deficiencies of one or more amino acids could have a wide range of deleterious effects upon an individual's health.

Many Americans, particularly children, teenagers, and the elderly, experience insufficient protein intake. This may lead to a condition known as negative nitrogen balance. Protein consists primarily of nitrogen, and, when the nitrogen level (in the form of amino acids) drops to a certain crucial point, negative nitrogen balance begins. This is manifested by a sort of cannibalistic state, where the tissues utilize nitrogen from muscles and similar "non-essential" tissues in order to return the nitrogen balance to normal. Negative nitrogen balance may also be caused by the consumption of large quantities of refined sugar. The typical diet followed by teenagers, children, and many elderly individuals may contain as much as one-fourth to one-half cup of sugar per day. Think about it. A can of pop contains six to seven teaspoons; a few cookies, another four or five teaspoons; a doughnut, another seven teaspoons; a hamburger with special sauce, ketchup, and fries covered with ketchup, three teaspoons (there is sugar in the bun, sauce, and ketchup); a chocolate malt, 8 teaspoons. Thus, in a typical person's daily menus it doesn't take long to accumulate a quarter or even half cup.

The primary problem with excessive sugar intake is that high-quality protein-rich foods are being displaced by the sugary ones. However, there is an additional insidious factor: sugar-induced protein damage. The refined sugar causes oxidative destruction of the amino acids within the body by a phenomenon known as *cross-linking*. Cross-linking is defined as a condition wherein cellular membranes become so damaged that they become hardened and stick together. Thus, the sugar is stiffening human tissues from the inside out. This stiffening greatly accelerates the aging process. It wreaks havoc upon the cellular proteins and membranes, altering them from their flexible fluid-like state to a stiffened and, therefore, malfunctioning one. In essence, the cell membranes and proteins become functionally incompetent as a result of excessive sugar intake.

Sugar addicts frequently have high uric acid levels in their blood. Uric acid is a breakdown product of cellular nuclear material. What is the implication? Sugar is killing human cells.

Individuals who receive a significant percentage (25% or more) of their dietary calories from refined sugar are at the greatest risk for amino acid deficiency. Cooked sugar is worse, because the caramelization process increases its toxicity. Additional high risk groups for protein deficiency include vegetarians and macrobiotic adherents. Their diets often omit the top sources of amino acids: meats, eggs, fish, and milk products. What's more, vegans are grossly protein-deficient. Often, their deficiencies become so extreme that they develop a swollen abdomen, a sign of serious liver damage. Incredibly, all such damage could be prevented, even reversed, by adding even relatively small quantities of animal protein to the diet.

The finest food source of amino acids is milk, which is a complete protein. Fresh milk, cottage cheese, and yogurt are the most readily available food sources for building a stable, healthy nitrogen balance. Unfortunately, tens of millions of Americans are allergic to cow's milk and/or products derived from it. However, goat's milk is an excellent alternative and is, in fact, more digestible than cow's milk. Yogurt is the most readily digested of all milk products, and the amino acids within it are efficiently absorbed into the bloodstream. Other excellent sources of protein/amino acids include brown rice, soybeans, alfalfa, spirulina, chlorella, and ground flax seed. Chlorella, spirulina, alfalfa, and ground flax seed are exceptionally valuable, since they are sources of raw (i.e. uncooked) amino acids. All these products are available in quality health food stores.

AMINO ACID TEST

Which of these apply to you (each response worth 1 point)?

1. mood swings
2. depression
3. anxiety and/or panic attacks
4. chronic fatigue
5. insomnia
6. weight loss
7. digestive disturbances
8. muscular weakness
9. chronic pain
10. impaired wound healing

11. heightened susceptibility to infection
12. diminished resistance to stress
13. nervousness and/or agitation
14. hair loss
15. slow growing hair and/or nails
16. brittle hair and/or nails
17. dry skin and/or hair
18. split ends
19. Do you drink one or more alcoholic beverages per day?
20. Were you a heavy drinker in the past?
21. Do you drink four or more cups of coffee per day?
22. Do you consume beverages or foods sweetened with NutraSweet on a daily basis?
23. Do you have a history of pancreatitis?
24. Do you have hypochlorhydria (low stomach acid)?
25. Have you had a portion of your stomach or intestines removed?
26. Do you have chronic anemia?
27. Do you have a history of panic disorder?
28. Do you fail to remember your dreams?
29. Do cuts or burns heal slowly?
30. Do you have reduced levels of protein in your blood (low BUN, albumin, globulin, creatine, etc.)?

Your Score _____

---

1 to 6 points *Mild amino acid deficiency*: Take digestive enzymes (2 or 3 capsules with each meal) as an aid to protein digestion. Increase the intake of protein-rich foods, especially highly digestible proteins such as chlorella, spirulina, bee pollen, eggs, raw nuts/seeds, and milk products.

7 to 12 points *Moderate amino acid deficiency*: Follow the previously mentioned advice plus take amino acids: 6 to 8 capsules of amino acid complex in the morning with a glass of juice (on an empty stomach). The sugar in the juice aids in amino acid absorption. An alternative would be to consume pre-digested protein supplements. Increase the dosage of digestive enzymes to 4 tablets/capsules with each meal. Eat fresh fish two or more times per week, since it is an excellent source of digestible protein. Add naturally-raised red meat to the diet: 3 or more servings weekly.

13 to 19 points *Severe amino acid deficiency*: Follow the aforementioned advice. Additionally, take 50 mg each of B-6 and zinc, since protein digestion and synthesis cannot proceed without them. Take an additional 3 to 4 enzyme tablets one hour after meals. Try the Protein Shake recipe. Eat a couple of handfuls of raw nuts every day. Add naturally-raised red meat to the diet: 6 or more servings weekly.

20 and above *Extreme amino acid deficiency*: Such an extreme amino acid deficit requires aggressive correction. Increase the intake of protein-rich foods such as raw nuts/ seeds, bee pollen, ground flax seed, eggs, yogurt, and alfalfa meal. Add naturally-raised red meat to the diet: a serving daily. Take the following supplements:

- zinc - 30 mg twice daily
- B-6 - 50 mg twice daily
- digestive enzymes - 8 capsules twice daily (on an empty stomach with juice)
- bee pollen - one teaspoon with breakfast and an additional teaspoon with lunch
- chlorella - 15 (tiny) tablets with breakfast and an additional 15 with lunch

Bioflavonoids

Bioflavonoids are a unique class of natural chemicals found exclusively in fruits, vegetables, herbs, and other plants.

Thousands of bioflavonoids exist in nature; so many, in fact, that it is doubtful that researchers will ever be able to fully comprehend or quantify them. What's more, each plant has its own unique combination of bioflavonoids. For instance, alfalfa contains more than 40 different bioflavonoids, each of which possesses a separate chemical function.

Recently, bioflavonoids have been intensively studied because of their anti-inflammatory effects, since they possess powers similar to many drugs. One group of scientists found that bioflavonoids, when combined with enzymes and vitamin C, perform equally as well as a commonly prescribed anti-inflammatory drug in reducing swelling, pain, and inflammation. Relatively few bioflavonoids have been thoroughly studied, and even with this mere glimpse of knowledge researchers have become impressed at their potent therapeutic value in the treatment of disease. Familiar forms are rutin, hesperidin, catechin, and quercetin. Some examples of foods containing therapeutic bioflavonoids include:

Blueberries: contain bioflavonoids, which prevent bruising, strengthen arteries, and enhance vision.

Cherries, strawberries, and grapes: contain a bioflavonoid (e.g. ellagic acid) which blocks the development of cancer and inactivates cancer-causing compounds.

Turmeric: contains bioflavonoids which reduce inflammation in the liver and aid in the treatment of liver diseases, including hepatitis and cirrhosis.

Ginger: contains bioflavonoids, which block inflammation in the stomach, intestines, and liver as well as aid in the healing of damaged tissues within these organs.

Alfalfa: contains bioflavonoids which reduce inflammation in the lungs and joints, which may prove useful in asthma, pneumonia, bronchitis, or arthritis.

Green cabbage: contains unique bioflavonoids which aid in the healing of internal ulcers, particularly stomach ulcers, and help prevent ulcer recurrence. Green cabbage juice is perhaps the most effective natural cure for internal ulcers. Other bioflavonoids in cabbage help block and/or reverse the toxic effects of nuclear radiation.

Citrus rind: contains bioflavonoids which reduce and/or eliminate inflammatory reactions in the joints. Citrus bioflavonoids also strengthen blood vessel walls and, thus, are effective in the treatment of nosebleeds, heavy periods, repeated abortions, bleeding gums, and easy bruising.

Bioflavonoids are found in all fruits, herbs, and vegetables. One method for determining the bioflavonoid content of a plant is the intensity of its color. Thus, red sweet peppers contain a greater number of bioflavonoids than green peppers, dark greens contain more than the light-colored iceberg lettuce, red onions contain a greater amount than yellow onions, dark bing cherries contain more than red cherries, etc. Additionally, fresh sun-ripened produce contains a richer bioflavonoid content than produce which is picked green and gas-ripened.

Recently, researchers discovered one of the most potent bioflavonoids ever. Known as resveratrol, this is the main flavonoid in red grapes. Resveratrol is a highly effective antioxidant. Its antioxidant properties are significantly more potent than either vitamin C or vitamin B. It is beneficial in the treatment of a variety of conditions, including spider veins, varicose veins, kidney disorders, kidney stones, easy bruising, bleeding tendencies, bleeding gums, liver spots, cholesterol deposits, back pain, arthritis, asthma, prostate problems, eczema, fibromyalgia, and inflammation.

Crude red sour grape powder is rich in naturally occurring resveratrol. This is made from mountain-grown sour grapes, which are naturally dried. This type of red grape is also rich in naturally occurring chromium and potassium. It is known as

Resvitanol powder, check health food stores or call 1-800-243-5242. Other excellent food sources of bioflavonoids include alfalfa, blueberries, turmeric, red peppers (sweet and hot), bing cherries, red cabbage, tangerines, oranges, grapefruit, lemons, limes, pomegranates, alfalfa, strawberries, raisins, and black currants. A high grade Mediterranean-source pomegranate syrup is available. For more information call the aforementioned number.

Black currants are one of the top sources of bioflavonoids. While high quality black currants may be difficult to find, an organic European-source black currant juice is available. Known as *Currant-C* it is currently only available by mail order: 1-800-243-5242. This is a super-rich source of naturally occurring bioflavonoids and vitamin C. When added to spring or carbonated water, this makes an excellent vitamin C and bioflavonoid tonic.

BIOFLAVONOIDS TEST

Which of these apply to you (each response worth 1 point)?

1. easy bruising
2. bleeding gums
3. nosebleeds
4. inflammation and/or swelling of the joints
5. swollen extremities
6. varicose and/or spider veins
7. heavy menstrual bleeding
8. retinal hemorrhages
9. repeated miscarriages
10. tendency to form blood clots
11. blood in the urine
12. hemorrhoids
13. glaucoma
14. fragile blood vessels (blood vessels which burst easily)
15. arthritis

16. fever blisters
17. petechiae (tiny red blood spots on the skin)
18. failing vision
19. blood in the stool
20. Do you have a history of coronary artery disease or hardening of the arteries?
21. Have you had blood clots in the veins?
22. Have you suffered a stroke, or do you have a significant family history of stroke?
23. Do you have a history of stomach and/or duodenal ulcers?
24. Do you avoid consuming fresh fruits and/or vegetables?
25. Do you consume aspirin, Motrin, or other anti-inflammatory drugs on a daily or weekly basis?
26. Do you suffer from shingles or genital herpes outbreaks?

Your Score _____

1 to 5 points *Mild bioflavonoid deficiency*: Take 1,000 mg of citrus bioflavonoids daily. In addition, consume foods and spices rich in bioflavonoids.

6 to 13 points *Moderate bioflavonoid deficiency*: Take 1,500 to 2,000 mg of citrus bioflavonoids daily. On a regular basis eat large helpings of fruits and vegetables rich in bioflavonoids. Take a natural crude bioflavonoid supplement, such as Flavin-C, four capsules daily. Also, eat the inside lining of citrus – the white pulp.

14 and above *Severe bioflavonoid deficiency*: A systemic deficiency of bioflavonoids increases the risks for bleeding disorders such as nosebleeds, easy bruising, bleeding ulcers, and petechiae (ruptured capillaries). Take a crude vitamin C/bioflavonoids supplement, such as Flavin-C, six or more capsules daily. Take also crude red sour grape powder, one teaspoon twice daily. In addition, take liquid propolis (non-alcoholic), 20 drops twice daily. Known as *Oil of Propolis*, this is the richest known source of bioflavonoids. Also take vitamin C; it works synergistically with the bioflavonoids to strengthen blood vessels and reduce inflammation (2,000 mg daily). Vitamin E helps obviate bleeding tendencies by normalizing blood clotting (take 1200 I.U. daily). Also, eat the inside lining – the white pulp – of citrus. Note: This is only true of organic citrus.

Enzymes (digestive)

Enzymes are complex protein molecules. They speed the various chemical reactions occurring within the human body. Incredibly, billions of enzyme molecules are synthesized every day by our bodies, primarily in the liver, pancreas, and small intestine.

Enzyme deficiency is extremely common in the United States as well as in other Western countries. In this syndrome the pancreas, the gland responsible for the synthesis of digestive enzymes, fails to produce the appropriate amount of enzymes for food to be digested optimally. This is largely a result of enzyme burnout from the prolonged consumption of processed and chemically contaminated foods.

Regarding the digestive process the pancreas synthesizes the vast majority of the enzymes. Unfortunately, pancreatic enzyme depletion is common in Americans and is largely the result of poor diet. Nearly 80% of the calories consumed by Americans today come from processed foods. Furthermore, there are well over 6,000 synthetic chemicals, which are "legally" added to food. This does not include pesticide and herbicide residues; the majority of commercial food also contains detectable levels of them. All such synthetic poisons disrupt enzyme synthesis. It is no wonder that pancreatic disease is common in America today. The pancreas is a delicate organ and is readily damaged by toxic insults. However, it may take a number of years before it finally collapses as a result of chemical toxicity, sugar overload, alcoholism, and/or nutritional deficiency.

A number of substances commonly found in the American diet induce pancreatic damage. These substances include coffee, alcohol, tobacco smoke, artificial sweeteners, food preservatives, food dyes, drugs, sulfites, MSG, pesticides, herbicides, and refined sugar. The latter is the most ubiquitous anti-pancreatic agent. A high-sugar diet causes a significant reduction in pancreatic enzyme output. The long-term ill effects on the pancreas are well known: hypoglycemia and, ultimately, diabetes—perhaps even cancer.

Diabetes afflicts millions of Americans, and hundreds of thousands of children and adolescents are included in its victims. Ironically, diabetes is entirely preventable by curtailing the intake of refined sugar early in life.

Sugar is only one of many culprits. Artificial sweeteners may in some respects exhibit an even greater degree of toxicity to the pancreas than refined natural sugars. Studies document that NutraSweet essentially stops the pancreas from producing enzymes. After only a few doses, the equivalent of that found in a half dozen cans of pop, enzyme production is fully obstructed.

A deficiency in digestive enzymes can result in a number of symptoms, most of which are related directly to digestion. However, digestive enzymes are involved in a variety of other functions, including protein synthesis, antimicrobial activity, and cellular cleanup, the latter being a sort of garbage collector/processor function.

Enzymes are found in all foods, but they are destroyed by heat. Thus, raw and lightly cooked foods are the only significant dietary sources.

ENZYMES (DIGESTIVE) TEST

Which of these apply to you (each response worth 1 point)?

___1. excessive gas
___2. fullness and/or bloating after meals
   3. poorly formed stools

4. constipation
5. greasy, pale, or gray stools that float
6. chronic heartburn
7. undigested food particles in stool
8. chronic diarrhea
9. colitis and/or irritable bowel syndrome
10. eczema and/or psoriasis
11. hives and/or other severe allergic reactions
12. lack of appetite
13. white spots on the fingernails
14. ridges on the fingernails
15. slow growing nails and/or hair
16. hair loss
17. stomach or bowel pain after eating
18. fatigue and/or somnolence after eating
19. rectal burning
20. arthritis or joint stiffness
20. Do you have hypochlorhydria (low stomach acid)?
21. Do you have a significant family history of diabetes, or do you suffer from diabetes?
22. Do you have a history of pancreatitis?
23. Do you consume on a daily basis one or more servings of foods/beverages containing artificial sweeteners?
24. Do you have a history of stomach or intestinal cancer?
25. Do you smoke and/or use chewing tobacco?
26. Is your diet high in refined sugar?
27. Do you consume alcoholic beverages on a daily basis?
28. Do you eat processed foods or fast foods on a daily basis?
29. Do you eat mostly cooked foods?
30. Do you avoid eating raw fruit and vegetables?
31. Are you a ravenous eater, or do you eat excessively fast?
32. Do you drink five or more cups of coffee per day?
33. Do you have mucous in your stool?

Your Score ___

1 to 6 points *Mild enzyme deficiency*: Increase the consumption of enzyme-rich raw fruits and vegetables. Take 3 capsules of papaya enzymes with all meals, particularly high-protein meals. Take also a non-glandular plant-based digestive enzyme supplement, such as Oregacyn Digestive Formula, with all meals, especially those consisting of cooked foods. Reduce the consumption of sugar, white flour, NutraSweet, and/or alcohol.

7 to 17 points *Moderate enzyme deficiency:* In addition to eating raw foods take digestive enzymes, zinc, and vitamin B-6. Both zinc and B-6 stimulate enzyme synthesis in the pancreas. Take 3 to 4 capsules of a digestive enzyme formula with every meal along with an additional 2 to 3 capsules one hour after meals. Or, take Oregacyn Digestive Formula, a combination of digestive enzymes plus herbal tonics, 2 to 3 with each meal. Curtail the consumption of NutraSweet and saccharin. Strictly avoid refined sugar as well as alcohol. NutraSweet greatly inhibits pancreatic enzyme production.

18 and above *Severe enzyme deficiency:* At this level of deficiency protein digestion and absorption is severely impaired. Aggressive treatment with digestive aids is indicated. In addition to the previous dietary recommendations follow this enzyme treatment regimen:

- With meals: 4 to 6 capsules of papaya enzymes and 4 capsules Oregacyn Digestive Formula
- One hour after meals: 3 capsules of papaya enzymes and 3 capsules of non-porcine pancreatin
- Two hours after meals: 2 capsules of papaya enzymes

Fully curtail the intake of refined sugar, alcohol, and NutraSweet. The latter greatly interferes with pancreatic enzyme output. Reduce the intake of cooked food, while increasing the intake of raw food. However, avoid the intake of large amounts of raw almonds, since they contain an enzyme inhibitor.

Coenzyme Q-10 (Co-Q-10)

Coenzyme Q-10 is one of the most unique of all nutrients. Technically, it fails to meet the criteria of a vitamin, yet, it is essential to life. When tissue levels of co-Q-10 fall to certain levels—25% of normal—death results. Co-Q-10 is produced in the body, but dietary intake represents a significant source. It is found widespread in foods, for which reason it was originally named "ubiquinone" (from the term *ubiquitous*).

One of coenzyme Q-10's main functions is the production of intracellular energy. In the case of humans the primary fuel produced on a cellular level is ATP, or *adenosine tri-phosphate*. This energy source is the basis of life, since all cellular reactions require and consume it. Thus, due to its role in energy production coenzyme Q-10 is of crucial importance for organs with rapid metabolic rates such as the heart, thyroid gland, adrenal glands, kidneys, pituitary, and lungs.

Coenzyme Q-10's role in cardiac function has received the greatest degree of attention among researchers. In fact, it was originally extracted from heart tissue (bovine hearts), the richest known source. During the 1950s and 1960s researchers discovered that animals which developed co-Q-10 deficiency died of heart failure. The hearts would enlarge in size, and the pumping power decreased dramatically. When the diets were supplemented with co-Q-10, the cardiac size and function returned to normal. The next step was to test the effectiveness of co-Q-10 on humans suffering from a similar condition: congestive heart failure. The scientists discovered that co-Q-10 worked equally well for humans with heart disease and completely reversed the pathology in a number of instances. Further research documented a powerful role in the treatment of hypertension, heart rhythm disturbances, angina pectoris, and coronary heart disease. In all cases the diseased hearts of cardiac patients, particularly those with congestive heart failure, showed a measurable decline in co-Q-10 levels from the norm. Co-Q-10 is also of exceptional value in the treatment of cardiomyopathy, a condition which leads to degeneration of the heart muscle.

A number of other organs/tissues become diseased as a result of declining co-Q-10 levels. These include the majority of internal organs, for instance the brain, liver, lungs, and kidneys, as well as visible organs such as the skin and gums. The gums are one of the most metabolically active tissues in the body and, thus, their need for co-Q-10 is exceptionally high. When co-Q-10 levels fall below a critical point, the gums degenerate. This is manifested by a lack of growth, recession, and an inability to adhere to the teeth. This recession causes the gums to become vulnerable to infection (pyorrhea).

Coenzyme Q-10 is similar chemically to vitamin E. The consequence of this similarity is perhaps best illustrated by the fact that many of the symptoms of vitamin E deficiency can be corrected by taking it. Furthermore, vitamin E enhances the function of the coenzyme. Thus, the two should always be taken in unison.

A number of other organs/tissues become diseased as a result of declining co-Q-10 levels. These include the majority of internal organs, for instance the brain, liver, lungs, and kidneys, as well as visible organs such as the skin and gums. The gums are one of the most metabolically active tissues in the body and, thus, their need for co-Q-10 is exceptionally high. When co-Q-10 levels fall below a critical point, the gums degenerate. This is manifested by a lack of growth, recession, and an inability to adhere to the teeth. This recession causes the gums to become vulnerable to infection (pyorrhea).

Coenzyme Q-10 is found in such a wide variety of foods that it is feasible to list only its richest sources: animal hearts and kidneys. Currently, virtually all coenzyme Q-10 available on the market is produced via microbial synthesis. This means that co-Q-10 supplements are a kind of natural extract rather than being artificially produced in a laboratory from petrochemicals. However, some of these types of co-Q-10 may be produced through genetic engineering. As always be certain of the quality of the source before purchasing.

COENZYME Q-10 TEST

Which of these apply to you (each response worth 1 point)?

1. muscular weakness
2. heart rhythm disturbances
3. delayed wound healing
4. enlarged heart
5. morbid obesity
6. chronic unrelenting fatigue
7. bleeding gums and/or pyorrhea
8. receding gums
9. high blood pressure
10. chronic kidney disease
11. increased susceptibility to infections
12. chronic gum infections (pyorrhea)
13. foul breath
14. muscular atrophy
15. accelerated aging of the skin
16. Do you avoid eating fatty fish?
17. Do you have a difficult time initiating weight loss,
18. Do you have an aversion/intolerance to exercise, or do you feel ill after exercising?
19. Do you have an immune deficiency disorder?
20. Do you have a history of angina pectoris and/or coronary artery disease?
21. Do you have a history of congestive heart failure?
22. Do you have asthma?
23. Do you avoid eating red meats and poultry?
24. Do you have chronic lung infection?
25. Do you smoke one-half pack or more of cigarettes daily?
26. Do you have shortness of breath after exertion?
27. Do you experience severe muscle pain, particularly after exercising?

Your Score _____

1 to 4 points *Mild coenzyme Q-10 deficiency:* Take 50 to 75 mg of co-Q-10 daily along with 400 I.U. of vitamin E. Avoid processed foods, especially refined sugar.

5 to 12 points *Moderate coenzyme Q-10 deficiency:* As tissue levels of coenzyme Q-10 begin to decline, the human body becomes vulnerable to the onset of rapid aging and degenerative disease. Protect yourself from rapid aging by consuming coenzyme Q-10 preventively. Take a minimum of 150 mg daily along with 800 I.U. of vitamin E. As a completely natural source of vitamin E and coenzymes take Pumpkinol, 2 to 4 tablespoons daily. Reduce alcohol consumption and avoid refined vegetable oils. Also, avoid the intake of cholesterol-lowering drugs, which aggressively destroy this nutrient. Strictly avoid the intake of processed foods.

13 and above *Severe coenzyme Q-10 deficiency:* Warning— severe coenzyme Q-10 deficiency may result in potentially life-threatening diseases such as congestive heart failure, asthma, emphysema, morbid obesity, and coronary artery disease. Take 200 mg of co-Q-10 daily. If you score greater than 18, take 300 mg daily. Eat beef or lamb hearts from organically raised animals cooked lightly (medium or medium rare) three to five times weekly. Avoid all dietary sources of refined sugar as well as refined and/or hydrogenated oils. The refined oils oxidize or "use up" the co-enzyme Q-10 found in the body. Be sure to take 1200 I.U. of vitamin E daily. As a completely natural source of vitamin E and coenzymes take Pumpkinol, 4 to 6 tablespoons daily. Additionally, if you have symptoms of congestive heart failure, asthma, or coronary artery disease, seek medical care immediately. What's more, avoid the intake of cholesterol-lowering drugs. These drugs readily destroy co-Q-10.

Carnitine

Carnitine is so crucial for human function that it should be deemed a vitamin rather than an amino acid. While many books describe it as an amino acid, it exhibits properties more like a vitamin, meaning that it is essential to life. In fact, Ensminger's nutritional encyclopedia describes it as vitamin-like. The deficiency is common in vegetarians, because this substance is found almost exclusively in animal foods. It was first discovered in meat extract.

Carnitine deficiency occurs both in slender and obese individuals. Vegetarians/vegans who suffer from distended abdomens are likely carnitine deficient. Thus, the deficiency results in liver failure. Neurological disorders may also result, since carnitine is required for delivering fuel to the neurons, that is the cells of the brain and spinal cord. Without carnitine the brain is incapable of processing fuel. Carnitine is also needed to transport critical fat compounds, needed by the brain for cell health. This is why mental fatigue, memory loss, depression, agitation, hostility, and mental confusion are so common in carnitine deficiency. The deficiency also explains many of the health problems faced by vegetarians, that is pale complexion, moodiness, anger, frustration, anxiety, apathy, fatigue, and exhaustion. In fact, strict vegetarians who suffer from obvious distended abdomens are probably carnitine-deficient.

CARNITINE TEST

Which of these apply to you (each response worth 1 point)?

1. eczema or psoriasis
2. heart rhythm disturbances
3. chronic fatigue
4. gum disease
5. muscles tear or injure easily
6. muscle twitching and/or cramps
7. spastic neck muscles
8. sluggish mental function
9. rapid aging

10. low HDL (good cholesterol)
11. heart flutter and/or palpitations
12. depression
13. heel spurs
14. calcium deposits in the joints
15. chronic arthritis
16. headaches during or prior to menses
17. high carbohydrate diet
18. eat mostly starches such as corn, wheat, pasta, bread, muffins, chips, potatoes, rice, etc.
19. difficulty losing weight
20. epilepsy
21. leg cramps
22. muscle tension or tight spastic muscles
23. heart pounds uncontrollably
24. get sick from exposure to cold damp weather or cold drafts
25. poor concentration
26. memory loss
27. poor endurance
28. exhaustion after minor exertion
29. high triglyceride
30. high cholesterol
31. slow recovery from exercise
32. dry skin
33. cholesterol deposits on the face (xanthomas)
34. rapid heartbeat without exercise (above 79 per minute)
35. muscular soreness, fatigue/exhaustion
36. muscular atrophy (loss of muscle tissue)
37. persistent abdominal distension
38. pale coloration of the face
39. chronic fatigue syndrome
40. highly intolerant to cold weather
41. gain weight rapidly/easily
42. Do you eat mostly processed or junk foods?
43. Do white flour products, such as bread, pasta, rolls,

noodles/macaroni, cookies, cakes, doughnuts, buns, muffins, lasagna, spaghetti, etc., constitute a large portion of your diet?

44. Do you have a history of angina and/or coronary artery disease?
45. Have you had a heart attack recently (within the past 5 years)?
46. Is your cholesterol level above 250?
47. Have you been diagnosed with an enlarged heart or cardiomyopathy?
48. Do you suffer from congestive heart failure?
49. Do you have a blood sugar level in excess of 200?
50. Are you currently taking anti-anxiety medications such as Prozac, Xanax, Zoloft, etc.?
51. Do you exercise vigorously on a regular basis?
52. Are you easily weakened by stress or physically intolerant of stress?
53. Is your blood pressure higher than 150/110?
54. Are you a binge drinker?
55. Do you have a history of kidney stones?
56. Have you had more than 3 kidney stones in your lifetime?
57. Do you consume candy on a daily basis?
58. Are you a soda pop addict?
59. Do you eat pastries on a daily basis?
60. Do you suffer from diabetes?
61. Have you been diagnosed with ALS, multiple sclerosis, or myasthenia gravis?
62. Are you involved in competitive or combative sports?
63. Do you suffer from Alzheimer's disease?
64. Do you suffer from Parkinson's disease?
65. Are you morbidly obese (over 30 pounds overweight)?

Your Score _____

1 to 3 points *Possible carnitine deficiency:* Carnitine is an amino acid, which is required for the metabolism of fuel in the body. Its role is to transport fatty acids, which are used for making energy, into the cells. After entering the cells the fatty acids are burned as fuel, a process which produces the molecular energy needed for bodily functions. A lack of carnitine essentially halts efficient energy production. This nutrient is found almost exclusively in animal foods. The animals synthesize it as a means of metabolizing fats. Carnitine is found in the diet primarily in the juice of red meat, a fact made evident by its name, i.e. carnitine from carnivore. Other good sources include poultry, eggs, fatty fish, peanuts, peanut butter, avocados, and cauliflower.

4 to 11 points *Mild carnitine deficiency:* A lack of carnitine impedes energy production, both in the brain and muscles. Even a mild deficiency may result in mental or physical fatigue. However, a deficiency of carnitine affects every tissue of the body. This is because this nutrient controls fatty acid metabolism, and the fatty acids are utilized by all cells. Fatigue is usually the first sign of carnitine deficiency, although mental sluggishness, weight gain, and memory loss are likely symptoms. Even a mild deficiency may cause a modest rise in cholesterol or triglyceride levels. To correct the deficiency take L-carnitine, 500 mg daily.

12 to 20 points *Moderate carnitine deficiency:* A moderate carnitine deficiency can impede the function of virtually every cell in the body. The liver, spleen, kidney, thyroid, and prostate gland are particularly vulnerable, since energy metabolism and fatty acid synthesis in these organs is carnitine dependent. Failure to correct the deficiency may lead to permanent organ damage. The heart fails to function properly in the event of a significant deficiency. Carnitine is found almost exclusively in animal foods. The animals synthesize it as a means of metabolizing fats. Carnitine is found in the diet primarily in the juice of red meat, a fact made evident by its name, i.e. carnitine from carnivore. Other good sources include poultry, eggs, fatty fish, peanuts, peanut butter, avocados, and cauliflower. To correct the deficiency take L-carnitine, 1000 mg daily.

21 to 30 points *Severe carnitine deficiency:* Carnitine is direly needed for fatty acid combustion. Without it, the cells within the body become infiltrated with fat and die, a condition known as balloon degeneration. The cells of the liver, heart, and kidney are particularly vulnerable to this damage.

Correct the deficiency by consuming carnitine-rich foods. The best sources are fresh red meat, juices of red meat, organ meat, duck, goose, chicken (with the skin on), and fatty fish, like salmon and trout. Peanut butter, cauliflower, and avocados are good sources. However, the type of carnitine found in meat is more biologically active than the type found in vegetation. Vegetables are a rather feeble, that is unreliable, source. Eat organically raised red meat at least once per day. Lamb is the best red meat source. Also, eat duck and goose as often as possible. Consume at least one avocado daily. Take supplemental carnitine, at least 1000 mg twice daily. Be sure to take the carnitine with a fat-rich or meat-containing meal. Do not attempt to correct the deficiency with supplements alone. Food is the ideal source of carnitine. Note: French duck should not be consumed. It has been discovered that the French feed ducks the residues from septic tanks, which are mixed by feed companies into the feeds. If buying duck, select organically raised types.

Taurine

Taurine is one of the most critical of all cell nutrients. An amino acid-like substance it is required for mineral transport. The fact is it is one of the body's most efficient means of transporting minerals into cells.

Taurine is a difficult nutrient to procure in the diet. Plus, it is readily destroyed by toxic chemicals as well as drugs. People who are on multiple medications are usually taurine deficient, as are those who endure prolonged hospitalizations. Individuals suffering from cardiac disease usually have a significant need for taurine. Thus, in the case of severe deficiency supplements are necessary.

TAURINE TEST

Which of these apply to you (each response worth 1 point)?

1. chronic fatigue
2. increased susceptibility to infections
3. lowered white blood cell count
4. accelerated aging of the skin
5. weak and/or flabby muscles
6. irritability
7. mood swings
8. muscle stiffness
9. muscle cramps
10. macular degeneration
11. tendency to form calcium deposits
12. agitation
13. psychotic tendency
14. spastic jerking of the limbs
15. seizures
16. low blood calcium levels
17. loss of peripheral vision
18. restless leg syndrome (legs become stiff or jerk at night)
19. spinal stiffness
20. angina
21. never or rarely eat whole milk products
22. history of one or more heart attacks
23. heart failure (congestive heart disease)
24. muscular wasting
25. light sensitivity
26. failure to thrive
27. high cholesterol level

28. consistently have light-colored stools
29. slow growing nails
30. never or rarely eat eggs
31. low cholesterol diet
32. sensitivity to cold weather
33. Do you suffer from epilepsy?
34. Do you drink alcoholic beverages on a daily basis?
35. Do you drink alcoholic beverages on a weekly basis?
36. Do you suffer from gallbladder disease?
37. Has your gallbladder been removed?
38. Do you suffer from heart rhythm disturbances?
39. Do you suffer from congestive heart failure?
40. Have you had a heart attack recently (within the past five years)?
41. Are you taking cholesterol-lowering drugs?
42. Do you take numerous heart medications on a daily basis?
43. Are you suffering from extreme mental stress?
44. Do you suffer from chronic liver disease such as hepatitis and/or cirrhosis?
45. Have you suffered from hepatitis or cirrhosis for more than 10 years?
46. Are you constantly exposed to chemical fumes?
47. Do you suffer from low stomach acid (hypochlorhydria)?
48. Are you following a low protein diet?
49. Do you try to get most of your protein from vegetables, grains, and beans?
50. Do you eat only small portions of meat, fish, or poultry?
51. Are you a diabetic?
52. Are you a vegan?
53. Are you a vegetarian?
54. Do you suffer from manic depressive syndrome?
55. Do you rarely or never eat red meat?
56. Are you consuming sugar or sweets on a regular basis?
57. Do you take mood altering drugs, such as Prozac,

Xanax, or Zoloft, etc., on a daily or weekly basis?
58. Do you take the tranquilizer drug Chlorpromazine?
59. Are you taking the antimalaria drug chloroquine?
60. Are you on intensive antibiotic therapy?
61. Are you vulnerable to severe allergic reactions?
62. Do you consume acetaminophen on a daily or weekly basis?
63. Do you have an enlarged heart or a condition known as cardiomyopathy?
64. On a daily basis do you take 2 or more medications?

Your Score _____

1 to 4 points *Possible taurine deficiency:* A lack of taurine may not initially be represented with obvious symptoms. However, to avoid a deficiency eat a more balanced diet that includes sulfur-rich amino acids. Taurine is found in relatively few foods, primarily breast milk, goat's milk, and organ meats. Small amounts may be found in red meat and eggs. It may also be synthesized in the liver, a process which requires essential amino acids, vitamin C, selenium, and vitamin B-6.

5 to 8 points *Mild but significant taurine deficiency:* Even a mild taurine deficiency can result in significant biological defects. Vision may be impaired and digestion upset. The immune system and hormonal systems may be disrupted. Taurine is needed for mineral metabolism. It helps transport them into cells. There, it helps fix minerals into the cells, so they may be more readily retained. This taurine-mineral complex is of particular importance in cells which must maintain large amounts of minerals such as the heart, brain, and artery cells. In this regard it is particularly important for the transport of calcium, potassium, and magnesium. Since the taurine-mineral complex is crucial for heart function, cardiac symptoms may result, even from a mild deficit. To correct the deficiency avoid all compounds which destroy taurine. If you are taking taurine-depleting drugs, see your doctor for advice. Avoid white sugar completely. Alcohol should be avoided. Eat foods rich in sulfated amino acids such as eggs (always with the yolks, because that is where the sulfur is), whole milk products, cheese, organ meats, and red meat. Taurine-rich foods are limited but breast milk, goat's milk, and organ meats are significant sources. To get at least the minimum amount of taurine eat red meat on a daily basis. Eat organic liver on a weekly basis. Note that foods rich in taurine are among the most complete and healthy foods known. Protein-rich foods from vegetable sources, like soybeans, rice, and grains, are devoid of this nutrient.

9 to 16 points *Moderate/significant taurine deficiency:* A moderate taurine deficiency can lead to chronic ill health. Illnesses associated with taurine deficiency include immune deficiency, chronic fatigue, macular degeneration, diabetes, congestive heart failure, heart disease, and epilepsy. Taurine is needed for mineral metabolism. It helps transport minerals into cells and helps the cells retain them. This taurine-mineral complex is of particular importance in cells which must maintain large amounts of minerals, like heart, brain, and artery cells. In this regard it is particularly important for the transport of calcium, potassium, and magnesium. Since the taurine-mineral complex is crucial for heart function, cardiac symptoms may result, even from a mild deficit. To correct the deficiency avoid all substances which deplete or destroy taurine, including alcoholic beverages and refined sugar. Prescription drugs destroy taurine, as do non-prescription drugs, particularly acetaminophen. Alcohol consumption must be strictly curtailed. Eat foods rich in sulfated amino acids such as eggs, whole milk products, cheese, organ meats, and red meat. Taurine-rich foods are few but include breast milk, goat's milk, eggs, and organ meats. To get at least the minimum amount of taurine eat red meat and/or eggs on a daily basis. If you are taking taurine depleting drugs, see your doctor. Strictly eliminate refined sugar consumption.

Avoid antibiotic-treated meats. Daily use of antibiotics should be evaluated by your doctor; seek to reduce antibiotic intake. Taurine supplements may be necessary; take 3000 or more mg daily. Note that foods rich in taurine are among the most complete and healthy foods known. Protein-rich foods of vegetable origin, like soybeans, rice, and grains, are devoid of this nutrient. Vegetarian diets result in the deficiency.

17 to 26 points   *Severe taurine deficiency:* At this degree of deficiency organ and/or cellular damage may develop. The individual may suffer a tendency for severe allergic reactions. Significant impairment of immunity is likely. Illnesses associated with taurine deficiency include immune deficiency, chronic fatigue, macular degeneration, diabetes, congestive heart failure, heart disease, and epilepsy. Taurine is needed for mineral metabolism. It helps transport minerals into cells and helps the cells retain them. This taurine-mineral complex is of particular importance in cells which must maintain large amounts of minerals such as the heart, brain, and artery cells. In this regard it is particularly important for the transport of calcium, potassium, and magnesium. Since the taurine-mineral complex is crucial for heart function, cardiac symptoms may result, even from a mild deficit. A severe deficit may readily result in vulnerability to heart attacks and/or brain damage or angina and severe heart attacks. To correct the deficiency avoid substances which destroy taurine. These substances include aspirin, prescription drugs, and alcoholic beverages. In particular, alcohol consumption must be strictly curtailed. Eat foods rich in sulfated amino acids such as eggs (always with the yolks, because that is where the sulfur is), whole milk, cheese, organ meats, and red meat. Taurine-rich foods are few but include breast milk, goats milk, yogurt, and organ meats. To get at least the minimum amount of taurine eat red meat and/or eggs on a daily basis. Strictly eliminate refined sugar consumption. Avoid antibiotic-treated meats. Antibiotics should be avoided. Taurine supplements are necessary; take 4000 to 4500 mg daily. Certain nutrients aid in taurine synthesis, notably vitamin C, vitamin B-6, selenium, and sulfur. For sulfur MSM, a common supplement, is an ideal source. Another major source is egg yolk. The daily consumption of three or more whole eggs provides sufficient sulfur for the body's daily needs. Take also selenium, about 200 to 400 mcg daily, since this nutrient boosts taurine synthesis in the liver. Note that foods rich in taurine are among the most complete and healthy foods known. Protein-rich foods from vegetable sources, like soybeans, rice, and grains, are devoid of this nutrient. Vegetarian diets lead to the deficiency, since there is no taurine in vegetation. Sulfur-containing vegetables help boost internal synthesis. High sulfur foods help replenish this amino acid. Eggs, milk, meat, organ meats, garlic, leeks, and onions are all high in sulfur.

27 and above *Extreme taurine deficiency:* This degree of deficiency may lead to severe organ damage and/or failure. The individual may be highly vulnerable to sudden or toxic allergic reactions, particularly to drugs. In fact, the individual who repeatedly suffers from toxic drug reactions is likely taurine deficient. The immune system is likely severely depressed. Visual disturbances would be expected and permanent visual loss likely. Taurine helps transport minerals into cells, and causes the cells to retain them. In this regard it is particularly important for the transport of calcium, potassium, and magnesium. Thus, it is crucial for heart function, and cardiac symptoms may result. An extreme deficiency may ultimately lead to heart failure and/or heart attacks. To correct the deficiency eat foods rich in essential amino acids and avoid all substances which deplete or destroy taurine. See your doctor about eliminating taurine depleting drugs. The primary drugs known to deplete taurine are anti-seizure medications, the anti-malarial drug chloroquine, the tranquilizer Chlorpromazine, and antibiotics. Alcohol destroys taurine and impairs the ability of the liver to synthesize it. Halt the consumption of all alcoholic beverages. Completely avoid the consumption of refined sugar.

Eliminate nitrated and antibiotic-treated meats. Eat foods rich in sulfated amino acids such as eggs (always with the yolks, because that is where the sulfur is), whole milk products, cheese, organ meats, and red meat. Taurine-rich foods are few but include breast milk, goat's milk, and organ meats. To get at least the minimum amount of taurine eat red meat and/or eggs on a daily basis. Strictly eliminate refined sugar consumption. Taurine supplements are necessary, take 5000 or more mg daily. Also, take additional amounts of fat soluble vitamins, since extreme taurine deficiency leads to biliary stasis. A lack of bile greatly impairs the absorption of fat soluble vitamins as well as essential fatty acids and carotenes. To correct this take vitamins A, D, E, and K on a daily basis. Take beta carotene, 25,000 I.U. daily. Also, take selenium, 400 mcg daily, since this nutrient boosts taurine synthesis in the liver. Note that foods rich in taurine are among the most complete and healthy foods known. Protein rich foods from vegetable sources, like soybeans, rice, and grains, are devoid of this nutrient. Vegetarian diets lead to the deficiency, since there is no taurine in vegetation. Sulfur-containing vegetables help boost internal synthesis. High sulfur foods help replenish this amino acid; eggs, milk, meat, organ meats, garlic, leeks, and onions are all high in sulfur.

Essential Fatty Acids

Fat is a subject of much research and discussion in the field of nutrition. Mostly, the term conjures up negative thoughts in peoples' minds. "Stay away from fats if you wish to avoid the major killers and remain healthy," we are told. While this may be true of certain fats, avoiding the essential fatty acids is dangerous. This is because these fats cannot be produced in the body and are required for the maintenance of the basic processes of existence. Without them, a variety of illnesses develop. The essential fatty acids are required for the synthesis of the cells of every organ in the body. In addition, hormone, protein, prostaglandin, and neurotransmitter synthesis are dependent upon essential fatty acids. A list of the ailments which have been associated with essential fatty acid deficiency includes:

- eczema, dermatitis, and psoriasis
- lupus
- seborrheic dermatitis
- hair loss
- heart disease and hardening of the arteries
- cancer
- alcoholism
- diabetes
- arthritis
- senility
- Crohn's disease and irritable bowel syndrome
- acne
- asthma and emphysema
- Sjogren's syndrome
- infertility
- adrenal insufficiency

A little-known fact is that when the weight of water is removed, the brain consists primarily of fat. It possesses a dramatic need for essential fatty acids in order to function normally. What's more, whenever tissues within the brain, spinal cord, or the peripheral nerves are damaged, the need of the nervous system for essential fatty acids multiplies exponentially. In fact, the need is so great that the body will essentially "steal" such fatty acids from other tissues in order to maintain the nervous system's requirements.

The saying that a person's brain is "shriveled up" may be literally true in the case of certain degenerative diseases of this organ, *many of which are caused by a prolonged deficiency of essential fatty acids.* The fatty acids are involved in moisture retention within the brain cells, and in the event of a deficiency a measurable reduction in the weight of the brain occurs. This is particularly dangerous in infants and children, who are highly susceptible to the deficiency.

Naturally occurring fats which are required for nervous system function include linoleic acid, linolenic acid, lecithin, EPA/DHA (abbreviations for fish oils), and cholesterol. Mental symptoms which may arise in the event of severe essential fatty acid deficiency include:

- attention deficit
- violent behavior
- mania
- memory loss

- autism and/or retardation
- anxiety/depression
- headaches
- seizures

Essential fatty acids occur in tiny amounts in a variety of foods. The richest sources are nuts, seeds, and certain grains, notably fresh whole wheat, barley, oats, corn, and rice. Soybeans are also an excellent source. However, the top food source is flax seed, which contains a high percentage of linolenic acid. This latter oil is difficult to procure in the American diet, which contains an excess of linoleic acid. Crude pumpkinseed oil (i.e. Pumpkinol™) is another superb source. Highly digestible, it is particularly effective for the reversal of the deficiency. Other excellent sources of essential fatty acids include the oils extracted from the seeds of the primrose, hemp, caraway, black currant, and borage plants. Walnut oil is also rich.

Food oils, such as those found in supermarkets, are traditionally regarded as top dietary sources of essential fatty acids. However, this is true only of those oils processed by cold-pressing methods. Commercial oils contain such a large number of contaminants and are so heavily processed that they can no longer be regarded as optimal sources.

An exceptionally high grade type of essential fatty acid supplement is available. EFA-Orega, it is a combination of wild spice oils plus berry seed essential fatty acids. Incredibly, the essential oil from berry seeds can be pressed, yielding a tasty, aromatic seed oil. This oil, being from a common edible source, red and black raspberries, is highly digestible and nutritious. The addition of spice oils offers an additional benefit, since the former act as preservatives. Therefore, the oil fails to go rancid. The latter is a significant problem with essential fatty acid supplements. Thus, in terms of a capsule EFA-Orega is the preferred type of essential fatty acid supplement. It may be readily given to children, since it has a sweet, berry-like taste. Currently, this is available only by mail order: 1-800-243-5242.

As mentioned previously regarding edible seeds pumpkin seeds are an exceptional source of fatty acids. Plus, the seed is a top source of vitamin E. Crude stabilized pumpkinseed oil (i.e. Pumpkinol) is a highly digestible source of essential fatty oils. Pumpkinol is highly digestible. Pumkinseed oil is highly vulnerable to oxidation, especially after opening. Thus, the stabilized variety is ideal. Pumpkinol is stabilized with potent natural antioxidants. It is the tasty, nutritious way to correct essential fatty acid deficiency.

ESSENTIAL FATTY ACIDS TEST

Which of these apply to you (each response worth 1 point)?

1. dry, flaky skin
2. dryness or cracks behind the ears
3. brittle hair and/or fingernails
4. acne
5. enlarged facial pores
6. growth impairment
7. dry or oily hair
8. eczema/psoriasis/dermatitis
9. chronic diarrhea
10. alopecia (patchy hair loss)
11. nosebleeds
12. bleeding gums
13. easy bruising
14. dry patches of scaly skin on the face and/or nose
15. patches of hair which are unmanageable (stick up on end)
16. split ends
17. poor or delayed recovery from injuries
18. intolerance to or slow recovery from exercise
19. delayed wound healing
20. tingling in the arms and legs

21. lips which are constantly chapped
22. attention deficit disorder (poor attention span)
23. asthma
24. loss of appetite
25. gritty feeling in or dryness of the eyes
26. irritability and/or nervousness
27. PMS (especially painful menstrual cramps, bloating, and/ or sore breasts)
28. sensation of dryness of the mouth and throat, especially when speaking
29. lack of tearing
30. obesity
31. unexplained weight loss
32. Do you take aspirin, Motrin, Indocin, Feldene, Naprosyn, or similar anti-inflammatory drugs on a daily or weekly basis?
33. Do you consume margarine on a daily or weekly basis?
34. Do you drink alcohol on a daily or weekly basis?
35. Do you consume refined sugars on a daily or weekly basis?
36. Do you have a history of repeated miscarriages?
37. Do you have Sjogren's syndrome and/or lupus?
38. Do you have emphysema and/or other chronic lung diseases?
39. Do you have Crohn's disease and/or irritable bowel?
40. Do you suffer from chronic joint pain (arthritis)?
41. Do you have a history of sluggish kidneys, chronic kidney disease, and/or bladder infections?
42. Do you have dementia, senility, Alzheimer's disease, and/or Parkinson's disease?
43. Do you have a history of ovarian cysts and/or fibrocystic breast disease?
44. Are you a diabetic?
45. Are you a tobacco smoker?
46. Do you have a history of prostate problems?
47. Do you take cortisone or prednisone on a daily or weekly basis?

48. Do you regularly use cortisone creams?
49. Do you have a history of infertility or impotence?
50. Do you follow a very low fat diet?
51. Do you take cholesterol-lowering medicines?

Your Score ____

---

1 to 8 points *Mild essential fatty acid deficiency:* Take 2 to 4 capsules of a berry seed oil source of essential fatty acids (e.g. EFA-Orega) daily. Use ground flax seed in recipes or as a topping on cereals, yogurt, or ice cream. Be sure to read all labels and avoid all foods containing hydrogenated and/or partially hydrogenated oils. These oils destroy the essential fatty acids.

9 to 18 points *Moderate essential fatty acid deficiency:* Take 8 capsules of EFA-Orega or primrose oil daily. Add to this 3 heaping tablespoons of ground flax taken in juice, milk, or water. Do not consume commercial oils of any type. Take supplemental zinc, vitamin B-6, riboflavin, and magnesium on a daily basis. As an excellent source of highly digestible essential fatty acids take crude pumpkinseed oil, i.e. Pumpkinol, three tablespoons daily. The latter is particularly effective at correcting the deficiency.

19 to 27 points *Severe essential fatty acid deficiency:* The consumption of alcohol and other substances, which destroy essential fatty acids, must be curtailed. Eliminate all refined sugars and oils from the diet. Consume only pure cold-pressed oils. Take 12 capsules of EFA-Orega or primrose oil daily.

Crude pumpkinseed oil is an additional source of essential fatty acids. The oil contains an excellent distribution of critical essential fatty acids, including linoleic and linolenic acid. It is far more digestible than flaxseed oil. Take 3 to 4 tablespoons daily. Additionally, take vitamin B-6 (50 mg), zinc (50 mg), vitamin C

(200 mg), vitamin E (800 I.U.), and magnesium (800 mg), since all these are required for optimal utilization of essential fatty acids. Lipase, a fat-digesting enzyme, is also recommended, that is for those who have poor fat assimilation. However, crude pumpkinseed oil is relatively easy to digest.

28 to 37 points *Extreme essential fatty acid deficiency:* Prolonged deficiency of essential fatty acids is a serious concern, since the function of all organ systems is dependent upon them. The earliest signs are manifested by skin disorders, since the skin is a barometer of essential fatty acid nutriture. As the deficiency deepens malfunction of the internal organs occurs, which may be represented by cellular degeneration, internal bleeding, and even cell death.

To correct this condition strictly avoid all dietary sources of refined, deep-fried, and/or hydrogenated oils. In addition, take 12 capsules of a berry seed essential fatty acid supplement (e.g. EFA-Orega), 6 capsules of lecithin, and 6 tablespoons crude pumpkinseed oil daily, reducing this after two months to 3 tablespoons daily as a maintenance. Supplement the diet with the nutrients necessary to stimulate fatty acid metabolism: B-6 (100 mg), vitamin C (2,000 mg), zinc (50 mg), magnesium (1,000 mg), vitamin E (1200 I.U.) Note: Most vitamin C supplements are derived from genetically engineered corn. For a completely non-genetically engineered vitamin C take Flavin-C, 6 caps daily. Natural-source vitamin C is far more effective than the synthetic.

38 points and above *Profoundly extreme essential fatty acid deficiency:* Prolonged deficiency of essential fatty acids is a serious concern, since the function of all organ systems is dependent upon them. The earliest signs are manifested by skin disorders, as the skin is a barometer of essential fatty acid nutriture. As the deficiency deepens, malfunction of the internal organs occurs, which may be represented by cellular degeneration, internal bleeding, and even cell death.

To correct this condition follow the aforementioned advice; strictly avoid all dietary sources of refined, deep-fried, and/or hydrogenated oils. In addition, take 20 capsules of a berry seed essential fatty acid supplement (e.g. EFA-Orega), 6 capsules of lecithin, and 8 tablespoons of ground flax seed daily. Supplement the diet with the nutrients necessary to stimulate fatty acid metabolism: B-6 (150 mg), vitamin C (3,000 mg), zinc (75 mg), magnesium (1,000 mg), vitamin E (1200 I.U.), and lipase (400 mg). Take also Pumpkinol, 6 to 8 tablespoons daily. After two months reduce this dose to 2 or 3 tablespoons daily.

Lactobacillus Insufficiency

Lactobacillus cannot be classified as a nutrient. However, it may be regarded as an essential dietary/nutritional component, since, like nutrients, a deficiency of lactobacillus can develop, and it can be taken supplementally. The term lactobacillus defines a family of bacteria useful in the maintenance of optimal health and the prevention of disease. Several types of lactobacilli exist, including Lactobacillus acidophilus, Lactobacillus bifidus, Lactobacillus caucasus, Lactobacillus salivarius, and Lactobacillus bulgaricus. These bacteria occur naturally in a variety of foods, although fermented milk products and sauerkraut are the richest sources.

Normally, these organisms are the predominant ones in the human intestine, existing in astronomically high numbers, several billion every few inches of bowel. However, in disease and general ill health their numbers decline dramatically. The fact is the vast majority of Americans suffer from lactobacillus deficiency. Why is the deficiency so common? Lactobacillus organisms are delicate creatures and are readily destroyed by noxious chemicals, particularly chlorine. Virtually everyone in the USA drinks chlorinated water. Chlorine is a potent oxidizing agent. In more familiar jargon it kills bacteria by "bleaching" them to death, leading to a gradual decline in bowel lactobacillus counts.

204 Nutrition Tests for Better Health

Secondly, antibiotics wreak havoc upon lactobacillus organisms. A single course of antibiotics decimates bowel microbes, killing the intestinal flora by the billions. This leads to the over-growth of certain organisms, such as Candida and others, which are resistant to antibiotics. The problem is that these organisms are pathogens, that is they are disease-causing. Antibiotics create this disastrous effect, whether taken in drug form or consumed in food. Thus, eating antibiotic-laced meats, milk products, fish, and poultry leads to an insidious decline in the number of lactobacillus organisms within the body.

The lactobacillus count in the bowel/vagina is a predictor for an individual's vulnerability to certain diseases. This is because these bacteria, descriptively known as the friendly flora, inhibit the growth of disease-causing pathogens.

Diseases associated with a deficiency of lactobacillus include:

- psoriasis
- eczema
- lymphoma
- high cholesterol
- hepatitis
- chronic candidiasis
- irritable bowel syndrome
- diverticulitis
- seborrheic dermatitis
- acne
- heart disease
- ulcerative colitis
- stomach acid
- intestinal parasites
- lupus
- colon cancer

Lactobacillus organisms are found in small quantities within and/or on a variety of vegetables, grains, and fruits. However, they are found in large quantities only in fermented foods. Top food sources include yogurt, kefir, kefir cheese, quark, tempeh, and sauerkraut. A special type of lactobacillus supplement is now available. Called Health-Bac, it contains four different types of naturally-occurring lactobacilli. These bacterial strains have been extremely researched and found to readily implant into the human gut. Health-Bac requires no refrigeration.

LACTOBACILLUS TEST

Which of these apply to you (each response worth 1 point)?

---

1. intestinal gas
2. bloating after meals
3. constipation
4. diarrhea
5. hard pebble-like stools
6. mucous in the stool
7. foul-smelling stools
8. hemorrhoids
9. easy bruising
10. recurrent nosebleeds
11. psoriasis and/or eczema
12. seborrhea of the scalp
13. indigestion and/or heartburn
14. persistent stomach aches
15. excessive rectal pressure
16. rectal fissure
17. less than one bowel movement daily
18. Do you take antibiotics on a daily, weekly, or monthly basis?
19. Do you often eat commercial meat, poultry, and/or fish?
20. Do you rarely or never eat fermented milk products?
21. Were you, as a baby, bottle fed instead of breast fed?
22. Do you have a history of chronic candidiasis?
23. Are you unusually vulnerable to the development of intestinal flu and/or food poisoning?
24. Do you have ulcerative colitis, irritable bowel syndrome leaky gut syndrome, or Crohn's disease?
25. Do you drink chlorinated water?
26. Do you have a history of diverticulitis or diverticulosis?

Your Score ____

---

1 to 4 points *Mild lactobacillus deficiency:* Increase the consumption of fermented milk products and yogurt. Eat at least one serving every day for one or two months. If you are allergic to milk products, take instead 2 capsules of lactobacillus acidophilus and/or bifidus with every meal. Or, take Health-Bac, 1/2 teaspoon mixed in juice/water either in the morning or before bedtime.

5 to 13 points *Moderate lactobacillus deficiency*: In addition to the yogurt take Lactobacillus acidophilus and/or bifidus supplements (1 or 2 capsules with meals). Curtail the consumption of commercially raised meats, opting instead for meats free of antibiotics and hormones. Avoid taking antibiotics, except for medical emergencies. Also, as an excellent source of Lactobacillus acidophilus and bifidus take Health-Bac, 1 teaspoon at night in a warm glass of water.

14 and above *Severe lactobacillus deficiency:* Consume large amounts of fermented milk products, for instance, three or four cups of yogurt daily. Also, take acidophilus and/or bifidus supplements, 3 capsules three times daily (with meals). Have your doctor take you off all antibiotics, topical and/or oral. Drink purified or mineral water instead of tap water or purchase a water treatment unit which removes chlorine. As an excellent source of acidophilus take Health-Bac, two teaspoons at night in a warm glass of water.

The Water Deficiency (Dehydration)

Water is the basis of life. Up to 75% of the weight of the human body is water. It is the most crucial of all nutrients for survival. A human being can live for weeks without food but only for days without water.

God made water. There seems to be no other conclusion. No human can make it. It originates from outer space. No one knows for certain how it happened nor precisely how it originally arrived upon the Earth. Yet, without it there would be no life anywhere.

Despite the fact that water is conveniently available in America, dehydration is just as common here as it is in many other regions of the world. This is largely because Americans often fail to make a conscious effort to consume water on a daily basis. There is another reason: essential fatty acid deficiency. The fatty acids act as a type of cellular glue, keeping cell membranes tightly fixed against each other. As such, essential fatty acids prevent excessive fluid losses, particularly from the skin. Individuals with severe essential fatty acid deficiency often become dehydrated, even if their fluid intake is normal.

There is yet another problem: water quality. Because of the concerns about water pollution and the toxicity of chlorine/fluoride, many individuals avoid drinking tap water, even though they might be thirsty. There is no simple solution for this dilemma. Keeping plenty of high quality bottled water available is one method that would prevent dehydration. Tap water purifiers are yet another solution for making water "consumable". Filtration drinking straws are another option. Some of these straws are capable of filtering up to 35 gallons of water and are ideal for use in traveling.

It is possible to consume too much water. In such an instance the body may be described as becoming "waterlogged". While relatively rare, the condition does arise occasionally in hospitalized patients receiving IV fluids. During my internship a surgical patient nearly died from water intoxication. She received an excess of IV fluids, which washed the electrolytes out of her body. The result was the patient developed seizures and slipped into a comatose state. She was subsequently "brought back to life" by infusing a concentrated salt solution.

Water poisoning also occurs in certain well-meaning fanatics. Such individuals often feel the need to "flush" poisons out of their bodies and may consume inordinate amounts of water— gallons—on a daily basis. Certain of these individuals consume purified water, such as distilled or reverse osmosis, which further depresses the electrolyte count. In one instance, a young woman saw me for a bizarre sickness. She had been "flushing toxins" from her body by drinking up to two gallons of distilled water per day. She was weak, light-headed, and panicky. Plus she complained of chest pain.The fact is, she was intoxicated—with water. Her heartbeat was weak, plus she had a severe heart arrhythmia. In fact, she was near death. I saved her life by injecting magnesium into her buttocks and halting her intake of distilled water.

WATER DEFICIENCY (DEHYDRATION) TEST

Which of these apply to you (each response worth 1 point)?

1. chronic constipation
2. hemorrhoids
3. dry mouth and/or eyes
4. dry skin
5. dry nasal membranes
6. dry or chapped lips
7. urinate 3 times or less per day
8. leathery skin
9. tendency to get shocked easily by static electricity
10. varicose veins
11. low volume upon urination
12 rarely or never eat salt
13. Do you suffer from chronic headaches?
14. Do you ever feel dizzy or lightheaded?
15. Do you drink large amounts of coffee (more than 3 cups per day)?
16. Do you drink large amounts of beer (2 or more beers per day)?
17. Do you avoid drinking water, and/or do you consume less than 2 glasses of water per day?

18. Do you drink large amounts of tea (3 or more cups) on a daily basis?
19. Do you take diuretics on a daily or weekly basis?
20. Do you have dark colored and/or foul smelling urine?
21. Do you have recurrent urinary tract infections?
22. Do you have a history of kidney stones?
23. Do you rarely eat fresh fruits and vegetables?

Your Score ____

1 to 4 points *Mild dehydration*: This condition is easily rectified; simply increase fluid consumption by drinking six to eight 8-ounce glasses of water per day. Avoid substances possessing diuretic actions such as tea, coffee, or water pills. Take two capsules of an essential fatty acid supplement daily.

5 to 10 points *Moderate dehydration:* Increase fluid consumption by drinking six to eight 8-ounce glasses of water per day. Additionally, take essential fatty acids: 8 capsules of primrose oil or unprocessed berry seed oil (EFA-Orega) daily. Avoid all diuretics.

11 to 15 points *Severe dehydration:* Warning—prolonged dehydration may result in damage to the internal organs, particularly the kidneys. Drink at least eight large glasses of water per day and take essential fatty acids: 12 capsules of primrose oil or EFA-Orega (crude, unprocessed berry seed oil) daily. Curtail the consumption of coffee, tea, and alcohol. See your doctor if you are taking diuretics and request that he/she reduce the dosage or preferably eliminate the drug(s). Also, increase the intake of natural salt, that is sea salt. This is because salt helps the body retain fluids, so they are not washed out through the urine.

16 points and above *Extreme dehydration:* Exceptional warning—prolonged dehydration may result in damage to the internal organs, particularly the kidneys. Drink at least eight large glasses of water per day and take essential fatty acids: 14 capsules of primrose oil or 2 tablespoons of crude pumpkinseed oil (Pumpkinol) or hemp oil daily. Curtail the consumption of coffee, tea, and alcohol. See your doctor if you are taking diuretics and request that he/she reduce the dosage or preferably eliminate the drug(s). Also, increase the intake of natural salt, that is sea salt. This is because salt helps the body retain fluids, so they are not washed out through the urine. Use sea salt in all recipes and foods. Eat a salty snack twice daily.

Section II

The Dietary Tests

Dietary Toxins

Many people think they are eating right, but they are not. For instance, some people believe that by substituting margarine for butter they are eating right. Others believe that eating pasta on a regular basis is eating right. Still others think that they can eat junk food, since they eat fruit, vegetables, and other wholesome foods on a regular basis. However, people with the latter attitude usually eat prodigious amounts of junk food.

Vegetarians believe they are eating right. Yet, as a result of such a diet they are usually deficient in a wide range of nutrients. In particular, vegetarians suffer from severe amino acid deficiencies. All cells require amino acids for growth. Vegetarian diets fail to supply the body's needs. Macrobiotic adherents are also convinced they are eating right, Often, such a diet is promoted as applicable to all. Yet, usually, its adherents suffer from a wide range of nutritional deficiencies similar to those seen in vegetarians.

In many Western countries in terms of the commercial food supply it is difficult to eat right. There is little good food in grocery stores. Organic produce is difficult to find in most regions. Instead, the food that is available is full of chemicals and low in nutrients. As a result, the majority of Westerners eat all manner of junk and devitalized foods. Are pastries, TV dinners, potato chips, cookies, crackers, white bread, deep-fried foods, preserved meats, canned vegetables, white rice, pasta, ice cream, pop, candy and similar nutritionally depleted foods still on your menu? All such foods are fully depleted. Thus, by eating these foods the body becomes depleted. Yet, these types of foods are the primary ones found in grocery stores as well as fast-food restaurants.

To prepare for the dietary tests I made several trips to the grocery store. There, I analyzed the ingredients of the various packaged foods, in other words, everything except fresh produce, milk products, eggs, and meats. These grocery store items were evaluated for their content of a variety of food components and additives. Remarkably, the majority of the food on supermarket shelves contained sugar. It is not the naturally occurring kind such as the sugar of an apple or the malt of a grain. Incredibly, of the 340 foods analyzed 255 contained added sugar. That amounts to over three-fourths of the foods surveyed. This can be readily confirmed by randomly selecting 20 items from the supermarket shelves and searching the labels for added sweeteners. At least half will contain sugar. The key is to recognize the names for its various forms as they are listed on the labels. In my survey corn syrup was the most frequent type, followed by sugar (beet or cane) and dextrose. Other types of refined sugars commonly added to foods include invert syrup, malt syrup, maple syrup, refined honey, glucose, white grape juice concentrate, fructose, and fruit sugar concentrate. Refined vegetable oil, a category which includes margarine, hydrogenated oil, partially hydrogenated oil, lard, tallow, and liquid vegetable oil, was the second most common category listed. Nearly one half of all supermarket foods contain such oils. MSG was a close third. Other food additives which are found in a large percentage of grocery store items include:

- white flour and rice
- corn starch
- synthetic iron
- coal tar dyes
- yeast and yeast extracts
- sulfites
- refined milk products
- nitrates and other synthetic preservatives
- ethylene glycol
- propylene glycol
- artificial flavors (derived from petrochemicals)
- caramel color

Hydrogenated Fats

Fats and oils are probably the most misunderstood, as well as maligned, of all foods. There is a general perception that if fats are derived from vegetable sources, they are health enhancing, while animal fats are toxic. As a result, it has been assumed that vegetable oils, even those which are highly adulterated, are safer to consume than animal fats of any type, including yolk of egg, pure butter, cream, and the fat found naturally in meats.

Ironically, in terms of saturation there is little difference between hydrogenated oils, such as those found in margarine, and the animal fats they are meant to replace, even though they are derived from vegetable sources. Here is why. Saturated fats are hydrogenated; that is the way they occur in Nature. This saturation explains why animal fats are hardened, that is they are solid at room temperature. In contrast, in Nature vegetable oils are liquids, that is until they are hydrogenated by the oil manufacturers. Thus, in summary, the terms hydrogenation and saturation describe the condition of the oil molecule. If a fat molecule is saturated, it is solid at room temperature; if it is hydrogenated, it is also solid. In contrast, if it is unsaturated, it is in a liquid state at room temperature.

You may want to try an experiment, the results of which are rather shocking. Take an egg poaching pan; put butter into one of the egg cups and margarine in the other. Bring the water under the cups to a boil and note the time that each takes to melt. Hint: butter dissolves almost instantly, whereas stick margarine will fail to fully dissolve, even after being subjected to the heat of boiling water for a full 10 minutes.

The consumption of hydrogenated oils has been linked with a variety of diseases, including heart disease, high blood pressure, hardening of the arteries, diabetes, multiple sclerosis, Alzheimer's disease, Parkinson's disease, arthritis, immune disorders, psoriasis, lupus, scleroderma, and cancer. Contrary to the position of the American Dietetic and American Heart Associations margarine is a cardiac poison. It is a major cause of hardening of the arteries as well as high cholesterol. In fact, recent studies published in prominent medical journals, such as the *New England Journal of Medicine*, document that margarine increases blood cholesterol levels to a greater degree than do natural cholesterol sources such as butter and eggs. What's more, it is a certain cause of cancer. The implication is obvious. Always opt for the natural over the synthetic.

HYDROGENATED FATS TEST
(each response worth 1 point)

Do you consume on a daily, weekly, or monthly basis:

1. margarine
2. commercial peanut butter
3. non-dairy creamer
4. imitation whipping cream
5. microwave popcorn
6. Egg-Beaters
7. imitation ice cream
8. Wheat Thins, Triscuits, Ritz, Waverly Wafers, Cheez Nips, Bacon Thins, or similar snack crackers
9. cookies
10. doughnuts
11. Twinkies, cupcakes, Suzi-Q's, Ho-Hos, and/or similar snack cakes
12. fruit pies
13. cinnamon rolls and/or other sweet rolls
14. frozen or restaurant pizzas
15. fish sticks or other breaded fish pieces
16. Tater Tots
17. French fries
18. breaded tenderloins
19. breaded or batter-fried shrimp
20. breaded chicken
21. tortilla chips
22. Cheetos or cheese puffs
23. corn chips
24. potato chips
25. gelatin molds
26. cakes (homemade and/or commercial)
27. imitation cheese
28. burritos/tortillas
29. artichoke hearts in oil

30. scalloped potatoes
31. tacos
32. tartar sauce
33. kid-style commercial cereals (Trix, Lucky Charms, Cap'n Crunch, Cocoa Puffs, etc.)
34. hot chocolate
35. muffins, including bran muffins
36. brownies
37. pot pies
38. pancakes
39. waffles
40. fondue
41. "broiled" restaurant fish (or chicken)
42. chewy candies (jelly beans, Juji-Fruits, etc.)
43. Pop-Tarts
44. boxed soup mixes
45. creamed soups
46. creamed frozen vegetables
47. graham crackers
48. pretzels (some)
49. Archway-style "home-made" cookies
50. Oreo-style sandwich cookies
51. peanut butter cookies
52. chocolate chip cookies, fudge, or chocolate covered cookies
53. crescent rolls
54. cheese cakes
55. bread
56. hamburger/hot dog buns and/or dinner rolls
57. cheese popcorn
58. Velveeta-type cheese spread and/or Cheez Whiz
59. ice cream cakes or sandwiches
60. puddings and/or pudding pops
61. egg rolls
62. pasta-style frozen dinners
63. frozen hash browns

Your Score _____

1 to 13 points *Mild hydrogenated oil toxicity:* There truly is no such thing as mild hydrogenated oil toxicity, since any amount is toxic. These oils are not meant for human consumption. They cannot be found in Nature and are produced strictly as a result of the manipulation of the chemical structures of naturally occurring oils. Avoid all dietary sources of these oils. Strict avoidance is necessary, because hydrogenated oils, even in small amounts, can cause cellular damage via the mechanism of lipid/peroxidation. The latter may be defined as the generation of rancid fats within human tissues. This may become manifested outwardly by aging of the skin as well as the deposition of unsightly brown spots, known also as liver spots. Certain nutrients, particularly vitamin E, beta carotene, bioflavonoids, glutathione, pantothenic acid, and selenium, help prevent lipid peroxidation. Spice oils also help prevent lipid peroxidation. Take Oregacyn multiple spice oil blend, 2 gelcaps daily. Also, take the oil of wild oregano, five drops twice daily.

14 to 29 points *Moderate hydrogenated oil toxicity:* You are consuming hydrogenated oils on a daily basis by the tablespoonful. If you continue consuming them, tissue damage will invariably occur. The cells of your body have no option but to attempt to utilize or absorb these distorted oils. As a result, the cell membranes become weakened or, more descriptively, they stiffen. This membrane damage leads to cellular malfunction, and, ultimately, disease may result. For instance, imagine a white blood cell with stiffened membranes; will it be able to catch up with an invader? Stop eating all foods containing hydrogenated or partially hydrogenated oils, and do not use margarine. Use butter instead. In addition, take the following supplements on a daily basis:

- EFA-Orega - 8 capsules
- vitamin E - 1200 I.U.
- beta carotene - 50,000 I.U.
- lecithin - 2 heaping tablespoons of granules
- selenium - 600 mcg daily
- ground flax - 3 heaping tablespoons daily
- glutathione - 300 mg
- vitamin C - 2,000 mg

Spice oils also help prevent lipid peroxidation. Take Oregacyn multiple spice oil blend, 4 gelcaps daily. Also, take oil of wild oregano, (i.e. oreganol) five to ten drops twice daily.

30 to 50 points *Severe hydrogenated oil toxicity:* You are consuming hydrogenated oils by the cupful. Carefully read all labels to ensure that absolutely no hydrogenated oils, partially hydrogenated oils, or margarine enter your diet. The question may arise as to what should be done about the hydrogenated and partially hydrogenated oils already absorbed into the cellular membranes as a result of years and/or decades of consuming toxic/hydrogenated fats? Drive them out of the tissues with the essential fatty acids and their vitamin co-factors. Take the following supplements on a daily basis for at least two months:

- EFA-Orega - 12 capsules
- lecithin - 8 capsules
- ground flax seed - 6 heaping tablespoonfuls (or two tablespoons of pure cold-pressed flaxseed oil or, preferably, crude pumpkinseed oil)
- B-6 and zinc - 50 mg of each (to aid in fatty acid metabolism)
- vitamin E - 1,200 I.U.
- selenium - 600 mcg
- N-acetyl cysteine - 1 gram
- glutathione - 400 mg

Spice oils also help prevent lipid peroxidation. Take Oregacyn multiple spice oil blend, 3 gelcaps twice daily. Also, take oil of wild oregano, five to ten drops twice daily.

51 and above *Extreme hydrogenated oil toxicity:* You are consuming hydrogenated oils by the tub full. Eliminate all dietary sources of these oils immediately. Follow the aforementioned recommendations for nutritional supplements. However, increase the daily dosage of vitamin E to 1,600 I.U. and glutathione to 500 mg. Be especially sure to take the spice oil extract, i.e. Oregacyn gelcaps, 4 to 6 caps twice daily for at least 60 days. Then, as a maintenance take 2 capsules daily. Also, take oil of wild oregano, ten or more drops twice daily. Additionally, eat restaurant food with caution; it often contains added oils. Be sure to ask your server to have the chef cook your food *oil-free*. Butter and pure extra virgin olive oil may be acceptable alternatives if the recipe must call for oil. Even so, the restaurant environment is a difficult one to control for the diet-conscious individual, since only chefs can provide a definite answer to the question of whether refined vegetable oils, hydrogenated fats, or margarine are added to the food. What's more, it has recently been determined that some chefs start with pure olive oil but dilute it with refined oils such as cottonseed oil. This practice is reprehensible. Cottonseed oil is one of the least edible of all oils and is, in fact, not even a vegetable oil. It is a waste product of cotton harvesting and is sold for no other reason than to stretch the profit dollars reaped by the cotton industry. In other words, cottonseed oil is inedible. Furthermore, it is usually contaminated with significant amounts of pesticide and herbicide residues, more so than any other type of oil. Therefore, if you must use olive oil at a restaurant, ask the chef if he/she dilutes it with any other type of oil.

There is yet another problem in many restaurants: butter substitutes. Under the guise of promoting good health, thousands of restaurants have switched from real butter to "Country Crock," "I Can't Believe It's Not Butter," "Promise," or similar butter/margarine substitutes. The servers often bring this vile mixture to the table whipped into a ball; it looks, smells, and tastes like butter. To make matters worse if you ask the server what it is, he/she will tell you that *it is butter, pure butter, nothing added and nothing removed.* The servers cannot be relied upon to provide an accurate answer, since they truly believe that the butter substitute is real butter. What's more, restaurant employees are unaware that margarine is inferior to butter as a food source. Thus, it is your responsibility to demand that the server ask the chef (or go back to the kitchen and ask the chef yourself; I have done this on numerous occasions) to check labels in order to be certain that this "butter" is the real thing and is free of all additives, hydrogenated oils, and margarine. Only then can you be assured that you will be eating the real thing.

Deep-Fried Food

There is a great deal of overlap between food containing hydrogenated oils and deep-fried food. Every year, billions of pounds of hydrogenated oils, as well as liquid vegetable oils, are used for deep frying food, both in restaurants and at home. These oils are also used in baking as well as in the manufacture of a wide range of packaged food. The distinction between this and the previous exam is that the deep-fried food listed herein may be defined as food cooked in a deep fryer, wok, pot, or skillet, resulting in the saturation of the food with additional refined vegetable oil, lard, and/or tallow.

DEEP-FRIED FOOD TEST (each response worth 1 point)

When dining at home or in restaurants, do you consume on a daily, weekly, or monthly basis:

1. French fries, home fries, and/or American fries
2. fried shrimp

3. fried chicken
4. onion rings
5. fried vegetable sticks and/or mushrooms
6. cheese balls
7. fried fish
8. corn dogs
9. chicken fried steak
10. chicken Kiev
11. breaded chicken breasts and/or chicken nuggets
12. Chinese food entrees
13. won tons and egg rolls
14. egg foo yung
15. stir fry
16. potato skins
17. omelets (not cooked in butter)
18. fried hot fruit pies and/or ice cream
19. hot Vienna beef and/or sausage (deep-fried)
20. fondue
21. doughnuts
22. Hush-Puppies
23. breaded tenderloins

Your Score ____

---

1 to 4 points *Mild deep-fried oil toxicity:* Eating any amount of deep-fried oils is too much. These oils are heated to incredibly high temperatures, plus they are used repeatedly. Essentially, these oils are cooked and re-cooked until they turn black, a process which astronomically increases their toxicity. Deep-fried oils are poisonous; avoid them entirely. In addition, take 800 I.U. of vitamin E daily to protect your body from rancid oil-induced toxicity. Also, take a potent spice oil-based antioxidant formula, such as Oregacyn, 2 to 4 gelcaps daily. Then, as a maintenance take one cap daily.

5 to 12 points *Moderate deep-fried oil toxicity:* You are consuming dangerously high amounts of deep-fried oils. The foods you are eating are coated and infiltrated with them. Cellular damage is assuredly occurring. Eating refined and hydrogenated vegetable oils increases the risks for cancer, heart disease, multiple sclerosis, Alzheimer's disease, Parkinson's disease, lupus, diabetes, psoriasis, and arthritis. These oils provoke inflammation and depress immunity. Eliminate all dietary sources of refined vegetable and deep frying oils and stop eating deep-fried food at restaurants. Take an essential fatty acid supplement, such as EFA-Orega, 6 caps daily.

Refined vegetable oils destroy vitamin E, and, thus, individuals who consume large amounts of deep-fried food are deficient in this nutrient. To correct this deficiency take a minimum of 1200 I.U. of vitamin E daily. Additionally, take daily dosages of the following antioxidants: vitamin C (2,000 mg), glutathione (300 mg), and beta carotene (25,000 I.U.). Also, take a spice oil-based antioxidant blend (i.e. Oregacyn), 4 to 6 caps daily for 60 days. Then, as a maintenance take 1 to 2 daily. Also, whenever cooking with oils, add a few drops of Oreganol and a few drops of wild rosemary oil to prevent oxidation.

13 and above *Severe deep-fried oil toxicity:* You are consuming deep-fried oils by the cupful. Stop eating these noxious oils immediately. It is likely that you are suffering from a sort of addiction to deep-fried food, a propensity which I call *The Hot Grease Syndrome.* The toxicity and tissue damage caused by these oils can be reversed by consuming large amounts of antioxidants and by permanently avoiding the consumption of deep-fried food. Take the following supplements on a daily basis in divided dosages for at least two months:

- vitamin E - 2,000 I.U.
- organic selenium - 500 mcg
- vitamin C - 2,000 mg
- beta carotene - 100,000 I.U.
- glutathione - 400 mg

Take also a multiple spice formula, such as Oregacyn, 4 gelcaps twice daily. After 60 days, reduce this dosage to 2 caps daily. In addition, take essential fatty acids: 6 tablespoons of ground flax seed and 12 capsules of EFA-Orega daily. Also, whenever cooking with oils add a few drops of oil of wild oregano and a few drops of wild rosemary oil to prevent oxidation. Plus, on a daily basis take the oregano oil (i.e. Oreganol), five to ten drops twice daily.

White Flour

White flour is found in thousands of supermarket foods. It is a subtle food additive. In other words, it is so easy to disguise that people are usually unaware that they are eating it. For example, are you aware that it is a primary component of creamed soups, including most of those served in restaurants? It is listed on food labels in various forms, including flour, white flour, wheat flour, bread crumbs, wheat starch, malt, and maltodextrin. What all of these forms have in common is the fact that they contribute unnecessary calories, while providing no flavor and minimal nutritional value.

All commercial white flour contains inorganic iron, which is added to it during the fortification process. The refinement and bleaching of flour destroys approximately 70% of its vitamin content and as much as 90% of its mineral content. During the refining of crude whole wheat kernels into white flour nearly 30 nutrients are depleted and/or destroyed. The only nutrients which are replenished are thiamine, riboflavin, niacin, and vitamin B-6 as well as iron. Recently, in some flour products folic acid has been added. Thus, white flour and the foods made from it, such as pasta and noodles, cannot be deemed nutritious in any respect.

White flour should be avoided for another reason: it is devoid of fiber. Because of this, it causes bowel disorders, particularly colitis, diverticulitis, and constipation. If you must eat flour, consume whole grain flour. The ideal is to purchase a whole-grain food processor and grind your own flour from fresh kernels. Such "farm-fresh" whole grains offer the following benefits, as contrasted to the whole grain products in the supermarket:

- they are free of toxicity; most whole grains are rancid by the time you purchase them.
- they are richer in vitamins and minerals than commercial pre-ground whole grains.
- they are easier to digest and far less likely to provoke allergic reactions.
- they taste better.

WHITE FLOUR TEST (each response worth 1 point)

Do you consume on a daily, weekly, or monthly basis:
1. crackers
2. pretzels
3. loaf bread
4. hot dog and/or hamburger buns
5. corn bread and/or Hush Puppies
6. rolls
7. Twinkies, Zingers, Cup-Cakes, Little Debs, and similar dessert cakes
8. doughnuts
9. cookies
10. chow mein noodles
11. canned soups
12. creamed vegetables
13. breaded chicken
14. breaded seafood
15. bread dressing
16. gravies

17. pizza
18. egg rolls
19. croutons
20. pasta-style TV dinners
21. spaghetti
22. lasagna
23. macaroni and cheese
24. canned macaroni dishes (Spaghetti-Os, ravioli, etc.)
25. French toast
26. waffles
27. pancakes
28. crepes
29. ice cream pies, cakes, or sandwiches
30. ice cream cones or drumsticks
31. cakes (commercial or home-made)
32. pot pies
33. burritos/tortillas
34. bagels
35. creamed soups
36. commercial cereals (cold)
37. commercial hot cereals containing wheat (Malt-o-Meal, Cream of Wheat, etc.)
38. malted milk and/or Ovaltine
39. muffins, including bran muffins
40. Pop-Tarts
41. broth soups with noodles
42. chunky soups
43. graham crackers
44. saltines
45. dumplings
46. croissants
47. tea or fruit cakes
48. breaded tenderloins

49. fruit pies
50. sweet rolls, including cinnamon rolls
51. candy bars containing cookies or wafers
52. pudding
53. batter breads (date-nut, pumpkin, banana, etc.)
54. flat or unleavened breads (pita, matzo, etc.)

Your Score ____

---

1 to 12 points *Mild white flour overload*

13 to 23 points *Moderate white flour overload*

24 to 34 points *Extensive white flour overload*

35 and above *Massive white flour overload*

At all levels of overload it is advisable to reduce white flour intake. Foods containing white flour are poor food choices. Ideally, bleached white flour should never be consumed.

Replace white flour products with unprocessed whole grains such as coarse whole wheat, oat meal, grits, whole rye, crude corn meal, brown rice, and wild rice. Alternative grains or grain-like foods include amaranth, teff, quinoa, spelt, kamut, and buckwheat. These may be purchased in health food stores and are less likely to provoke allergic reactions than the more common grains.

White flour is inedible, because it is devoid of nutrients. Its fiber is stripped away, its vitamins are destroyed by refining and bleaching, and its minerals are almost entirely removed. Those who score in the extensive or massive category have an additional concern: inorganic iron toxicity. That is because all white flour and white flour products are fortified with iron as iron sulfate, a chemical form little different from iron filings. When ingested over a prolonged period, inorganic iron may cause liver damage and also increase the risk for heart disease and cancer.

Some of the most valuable scientific studies on iron toxicity in humans were performed by Richard G. Stevens, Ph.D. His monumental research, which was published in the *American Journal of Clinical Nutrition,* documented as much as a three-fold increased risk for these diseases, depending upon the degree of elevation in the iron levels. These figures apply only to men and post-menopausal women, both of whom have low nutritional requirements for iron. Since it is difficult to eliminate via the normal excretory pathways, iron readily accumulates within the tissues. Thus, men and post-menopausal women should curtail the consumption of grains fortified with inorganic iron, and that means all foods containing white flour and rice, including pasta.

White flour is pure starch. This starch consists molecu-larly of sugar molecules attached by chemical bonds. Once ingested, the starch of white flour is rapidly broken down into glucose. In sedentary individuals the glucose is poorly utilized and is usually converted into triglycerides or fat. Thus, the consumption of white flour products is a contributing factor in causing blood sugar disturbances, obesity, high triglycerides, and high cholesterol as well as heart disease itself.

Pasta

Pasta has been touted as a health food, particularly over the last 20 years. Currently, it is hailed as the ideal replacement for traditional dishes such as meat, fish, and poultry. This is primarily because of its low fat content.

There is a certain degree of overlap between this exam and the previous one, since pasta is made from white flour. Yet, it serves to emphasize a point; commercial pasta is merely white flour molded into a variety of shapes. It is just as nutritionally defective as eating white bread and is one of the major sources for the ingestion of inorganic iron in the American diet.

228 Nutrition Tests for Better Health

PASTA TEST (each response worth 1 point)

Do you consume on a daily or weekly basis:
1. soup with noodles, pasta shells, or "alphabets"
2. spaghetti
3. pasta dishes and/or entrees in restaurants
4. hamburger helper and/or similar products
5. salads containing pasta
6. Spaghettios or goulash
7. ravioli
8. macaroni and cheese
9. pasta-style TV dinners
10. lasagna
11. linguine

Your Score ____

Any score means you are consuming an excess of pasta. Pasta offers no significant nutritional value in terms of vitamins and minerals. In addition, it contains inorganic iron, which destroys vitamins A, C, E, and K.

Spinach, soy, and whole wheat pasta provide a wider range of nutrients than the standard commercial types. However, the difference is not significant; vitamins and minerals are found scattered in commercial grain flours in trace amounts. If the objective is to consume nutrient-dense foods, pasta is a poor choice. For as many calories as it contains and as much poundage as it can put on, superior food selections can be made in the quest to eat nutritionally.

Certainly, Americans love eating grains. In fact, millions of Americans are addicted to them, this being largely the result of food allergy. Even so, whole grains, if fresh and properly prepared, are relatively good sources of vitamins and minerals. Plus, they are loaded with fiber. Barring food allergy there is usually no need to give grains up forever. Just eat them judiciously. Plus, emphasize alternative grains such as spelt, kamut, teff, oat bran, rice bran, and quinoa.

Refined Milk Products

Pure unprocessed milk is a wholesome food, just as is whole wheat. However, like wheat, milk can be refined to such a degree that its nutritional value is disrupted or destroyed. The primary concern in milk adulteration is homogenization, a process which alters the natural chemistry of the milk. Homogenization breaks milk's naturally large fat globules into microscopically tiny globules. These globules are absorbed directly into the bloodstream and fail to undergo the natural digestive processes necessary to render them non-toxic. While unprocessed whole milk, despite its fat content, is a safe food, evidence exists that the consumption of large quantities of homogenized milk may contribute to heart disease. So, don't overdo it. What's more, select organic whole milk products instead of the commercial types, which may be contaminated with bovine growth hormone.

Skim and non-fat dry milk are the primary types of refined milk products used as food additives. Other refined milk derivatives commonly found in processed foods include calcium caseinate (or casein), milk solids, whey, butter solids, and caramel coloring.

REFINED MILK PRODUCTS TEST
(each response worth 1 point)

Do you consume on a daily or weekly basis:
1. reduced fat ice cream
2. ice milk (swirl cones, Dairy Queen, etc.)

3. puddings and/or custards
4. coffee creamers
5. non-fat dry milk
6. evaporated or condensed milk
7. skim or one percent milk
8. Cheetos, Cheez Nips, cheese popcorn, or similar snacks
9. skim milk (hard) cheeses
10. low-fat cottage cheese
11. fudgesicles, froststicks, Bon Bons, Drumsticks, Eskimo Pies, Dove bars, or similar products
12. artificial cream or eggs
13. artificial ice cream
14. Velveeta, Cheez Whiz, and/or similar processed cheese products
15. processed American cheese
16. hot chocolate
17. creamed vegetables
18. creamed soups
19. gravies
20. cookies (some)
21. yogurt (non-fat or low-fat)
22. artificial sour cream
23. processed cheese dip
24. nachos or cheese tortilla chips
25. caramels and/or taffy
26. chocolate coated candy bars and/or chocolates
27. Do you drink 3 or more glasses of non-fat or 1% milk daily?
28. Do you consume foods containing caramel coloring?

Your Score _____

1 to 7 points *Mild refined milk overload*
8 to 14 points *Moderate refined milk overload*
15 and above *Severe refined milk overload*

The advice for all these categories is the same: avoid processed milk products and/or foods containing them. As an alternative select fresh milk products made from whole milk. Use cream instead of coffee creamer. Instead of skim or 1% milk drink organic whole cow's milk. However, for the majority of adults it is advisable to keep the milk consumption at two glasses or less daily, unless you have access to certified non-homogenized milk. If you are sensitive to cow's milk, use goat's milk, which is easier to digest and less allergenic than cow's milk. There are a number of non-homogenized (but pasteurized) goats milk products available. If taken in small amounts these may be well tolerated by milk-sensitive individuals. In some illnesses milk consumption is crucial. Examples include severe protein deficiency, wasting diseases, failure to thrive, and tuberculosis. These wasting diseases create a constant demand upon amino acid stores. Thus, a source of highly absorbable amino acids is required. This is why milk is of value. Its amino acids are thoroughly absorbed after ingestion.

Certain individuals are intolerant to all types of milk. Many of these individuals suffer from a condition known as *lactose intolerance*. Rather than being an allergy, this condition is due to a deficiency of the enzyme required for breaking lactose (i.e. milk sugar) into its component parts. The unabsorbed lactose irritates the intestines, causing bloating, cramps, indigestion, and/or diarrhea. Lactose intolerance can be corrected simply by taking capsules of the missing enzyme, *lactase*, whenever consuming milk products. However, allergy to milk products is relatively common in the United States. Thus, even fresh whole milk products are unacceptable food sources for certain individuals.

Chemical contamination of milk is another concern. Dairy cattle are routinely administered antibiotics. They may also be dipped or sprayed with pesticides. Hormones and other drugs are frequently given. Of perhaps greater concern is the FDA's approval of bovine growth hormone. This is used to force cows to produce larger volumes of milk. It offers no health benefits, rather, it detracts from health. The fact is the safety of this hormone is dubious. Evidence links its use to growth disturbances in children as well as tumor development. Eventually, it will be proven to be a human carcinogen.

Yeast-in-Foods

Yeasts are added to foods for several reasons. They are leavening agents. They are also added to enhance flavor. Additionally, they are sources of nutrients, notably B-complex vitamins and protein.

Virtually all baked goods contain yeast, and this is particularly true of breads, buns, muffins, rolls, cakes, and doughnuts. The rule of thumb is that if it is raised and/or has a crust, it contains yeast. A variety of terms are used for describing yeast additives on food labels, including:

- autolyzed yeast protein
- hydrolyzed vegetable protein
- vegetable protein
- bakers yeast
- brewers and torula yeast

Fermented foods and beverages are another major source of yeasts. This is because yeasts are commonly used as starters for fermented foods, or they may multiply within the foods as a result of the fermentation process. Such foods and beverages include baked goods, alcoholic beverages (particularly wine and beer), vinegar, soy sauce, and cheese.

Yeasts are toxic only to people who are sensitive to them. Allergy to yeasts may result in a variety of symptoms, including rashes, vaginitis, colitis, asthma, intestinal gas, bloating, indigestion, cold/flu syndromes, sinusitis, painful joints, and migraine headaches.

YEAST-IN-FOODS TEST (each response worth 1 point)

Do you consume on a daily, weekly, or monthly basis:

1. bagels
2. crackers
3. cookies
4. pretzels
5. pancakes and/or waffles
6. cracker crumbs and/or croutons
7. dry roasted nuts (some)
8. breaded foods
9. canned soups (some)
10. TV dinners
11. bologna
12. breakfast strips
13. ravioli
14. noodles and/or lasagna
15. pizza
16. Sloppy Joe mix
17. broth soups and/or bouillon
18. protein powders
19. boxed soup mixes
20. breads (including pita bread)
21. hamburger and/or hot dog buns
22. dinner rolls, muffins and/or croissants
23. soy sauce (some)
24. egg rolls
25. sweet rolls, cake, and/or doughnuts
26. pasta-style TV dinners
27. breaded fish and seafood
28. aged cheeses
29. horseradish
30. pot pies
31. root beer

32. vitamin tablets containing yeast
33. alcoholic beverages, particularly beers and wines
34. vinegar
35. batter cakes (date-nut, pumpkin, banana, etc.)

Your Score _____

---

1 to 9 points   *Mild dietary yeast overload*
10 to 19 points   *Moderate dietary yeast overload*
20 to 28 points   *Severe dietary yeast overload*
29 and above   *Extreme dietary yeast overload*

For each of these categories the advice is the same: reduce the consumption of yeast-containing foods. This is particularly true for individuals who have a history of multiple food allergies. Such individuals are often allergic to dietary yeasts and may suffer violent reactions upon ingesting foods containing them. Thus, those who suffer from allergy-induced diseases, such as candidiasis, hives, bronchitis, asthma, arthritis, colitis, eczema, sinusitis, mental illness, ear infections, and migraine headaches, are likely to significantly benefit from a yeast-free diet. In particular, asthmatics, who score high on this exam (above 20), are likely to achieve a rapid improvement if dietary sources of yeasts are thoroughly eliminated.

Inorganic Iron

This test covers essentially the same material as the white flour and pasta tests. However, it is included to emphasize a point; many Americans are unknowingly consuming vast amounts of inorganic iron. Since iron is one of the few nutrients which steadily accumulates in the body and since it is potentially toxic, it is important that people know where they stand in terms of iron intake.

For every 10% increase in tissue iron stores above normal the risk for certain diseases, notably heart disease, arthritis, and cancer, is nearly doubled. Thus, in many individuals the intake of inorganic iron should be restricted, just as the consumption of MSG, sulfites, sugar, and caffeine should be eliminated or reduced. Men, as well as post-menopausal women with normal blood counts, should significantly reduce their consumption of foods fortified with inorganic iron. What's more, they should never take supplements containing it. Such individuals usually receive all the iron they need from consuming foods naturally rich in this nutrient such as red meats, eggs, and spinach.

Medically, iron toxicity is known by the terms *hemosiderosis* and *hemochromatosis*. The distinction between these two conditions is primarily the fact that the latter is a more serious illness, involving a greater degree of iron deposition within critical internal organs. Both are associated with toxic accumulations of iron in a wide range of tissues, including the skin, mucous membranes, liver, spleen, lymph glands, pancreas, joints, pituitary, and heart.

Hemosiderosis and hemochromatosis are difficult to diagnose based upon clinical presentation alone. That is because the symptoms are often vague and are commonly observed in a variety of other conditions. However, by combining symptom evaluation with a thorough blood analysis, the diagnosis can be readily determined. Symptoms of iron toxicity include weakness, severe fatigue, loss of appetite, abdominal pain, chronic infection, diarrhea, nausea, and weight loss. In addition, iron toxicity may initially present with the classic symptoms of diabetes: weight loss, fatigue, excessive thirst, and frequent urination. This is due to the fact that the excess iron causes destruction of the pancreas, specifically those cells responsible for the synthesis of insulin.

Excessive iron accumulation may not be due exclusively to increased iron intake. It may be the result of a genetic defect in iron metabolism/absorption. Individuals with the defective gene absorb iron at an accelerated rate, as much as ten times normal. Researchers have discovered that iron absorption can be blocked by consuming megadoses of certain minerals such as calcium, magnesium, silicon, and zinc.

The existence of iron overload can be confirmed by blood testing. If you scored high on this exam, be sure to see your doctor and request that the appropriate tests be performed. Only then can you be certain that iron toxicity exists.

INORGANIC IRON TEST (each response worth 1 point)

Do you consume on a daily or weekly basis:

1. pasta
2. bread (pita, leavened, unleavened)
3. hot dog and/or hamburger buns
4. dinner rolls and/or croissants
5. creamed vegetables
6. muffins
7. bagels
8. sweet rolls and/or doughnuts
9. burritos and tortillas
10. cupcakes, Twinkies, Suzi Qs, or similar desserts
11. red meats (a rich source of organic iron)
12. cookies
13. cakes and/or pies
14. waffles and/or pancakes
15. Pop-Tarts
16. pretzels
17. creamed soups
18. commercial cereals (most)
19. Malt-O-Meal, Cream of Wheat, and/or similar hot cereals containing wheat
20. malted milk
21. croutons
22. brownies
23. boxed or canned soups with noodles
24. multiple-vitamins containing iron

25. Have you received numerous blood transfusions (8 or more)?
26. Do you have a history of an elevated red blood cell count (polycythemia or leukemia)?
27. Do you drink red wines on a daily or weekly basis?
28. Do you cook in an iron skillet often?
29. Do you take iron pills or Geritol, even though you are not anemic?

Your Score _____

1 to 7 points *Mild iron toxicity:* Inorganic iron, even in relatively small amounts, may provoke tissue damage. Men don't need the extra iron. Avoid all foods fortified with iron. Vitamins containing iron should also be avoided. Iron-free multiple vitamins are available at many health food stores.

8 to 15 points *Moderate iron toxicity:* At this level of iron overload tissue damage is likely to occur. Further accumulation may significantly increase the risks for degenerative diseases such as diabetes, arthritis, lupus, multiple sclerosis, hardening of the arteries, heart disease, and cancer. Follow the previously mentioned advice, being particularly careful to avoid all iron-fortified foods. Take an iron-free multiple mineral tablet as an aid to blocking iron absorption. Increase the consumption of calcium-rich foods, since this mineral is the most effective one for preventing iron absorption. To flush excessive iron from the tissues take Gene's wild greens, five dropperfuls twice daily (Note this is only available via mail-order: 1-800-243-5242).

16 to 22 points *Severe iron toxicity:* Adhere to the previously mentioned advice, being sure to carefully check all food labels for added iron. In addition, strictly avoid alcohol consumption, since it markedly increases iron absorption. Blood tests for iron overload are indicated. Supplement the diet on a daily basis with a multiple-mineral (iron-free) in addition to 1,000 mg of calcium. Consider blood-letting, i.e. therapeutic phlebotomy, as a cure. See your doctor about removing one pint bimonthly until iron levels normalize. To flush excessive iron from the tissues take Gene's wild greens, five dropperfuls twice daily (this is only available via mail-order: 1-800-243-5242.

23 and above *Extreme iron toxicity:* Warning—at this level of iron intake the risks for a variety of degenerative diseases, including cancer, arthritis, heart disease, lung disease, Alzheimer's disease, lupus, diabetes, multiple sclerosis, and liver disease, are greatly increased. Follow the previously mentioned advice, strictly avoiding all dietary sources of iron. In addition, take the following minerals on a daily basis: calcium (2,000 mg), zinc (60 mg), magnesium (1,000 mg), and silica (2,000 mg). To flush excessive iron from the tissues take Gene's Wild Greens, five to ten droppers full twice daily (this is only available via mail-order: 1-800-243-5242). Consider bloodletting, i.e. therapeutic phlebotomy, as a cure. Under a doctor's care one pint per month may be removed until iron levels normalize.

In extreme cases of iron overload food sources of iron, such as red meat, spinach, red wine, prunes, and raisins, must also be reduced or eliminated. In particular, the elimination of all sources of white flour is desirable. See your doctor and request blood tests for iron overload, including serum iron and ferritin levels. If the ferritin level is excessively high (above 200), therapeutic phlebotomy may be necessary. Levels above 350 may be an early signal of internal malignancy.

Refined Sugar

The majority of commercial foods available in America are laced with refined sugars. These sugars, which include white sugar, corn syrup, glucose, dextrose, and fructose, are the most commonly used of all food additives. In fact, they are so commonly found in food that the consumption of refined sugars in America exceeds 150 pounds per person per year. That is an incredibly large amount of sugar to be ingesting. Just imagine; it amounts to the consumption of more than a ten-pound bag of white sugar by every American woman, man, or child.

Refined sugars are found in an inordinate number of commercial foods. Regardless of their forms or names all refined sugars react within the body in a similar manner. In other words, there is predictable damage which results from such extensive consumption. Sugar depletes the body of a wide range of vitamins and minerals. It also dependably destroys the glands, especially the adrenal glands.

The dilemma is that the sugar offers no nutritional value, being devoid of all traces of vitamins, minerals, enzymes, and proteins. Thus, it causes the consumption of nutrients. Nutrients aggressively destroyed by refined sugar include B-vitamins, zinc, magnesium, calcium, essential fatty acids, and vitamin C. It also causes the oxidation, that is destruction, of protein.

Hidden sugar creates a wide array of health problems. Both physical and mental symptoms often result from the consumption of disguised sugar. Of perhaps greater concern is the rising incidence of diseases directly related to sugar consumption: diabetes, stroke, cancer, senility, arthritis, hypertension, schizophrenia, and heart disease. What's more, in children and adolescents, many of these diseases are developing at an alarming frequency. Today, incredibly, children are suffering from high cholesterol as well as diabetes, which are also commonly developing in teenagers. Even heart disease is far from rare in these groups.

In children, adolescents, and adults scientific studies correlate the consumption of refined sugar with the rising incidence of heart disease, hardening of the arteries, high cholesterol, behavioral disorders, learning deficit, blood sugar disorders, obesity, and diabetes Does it make sense to perpetuate this problem by continually feeding the youth sugar-infested foods?

In many respects adults, particularly the elderly, exhibit an even greater vulnerability to the noxious effects of refined sugar than do children. Sugar increases cholesterol and triglyceride counts, damages arterial linings, raises blood pressure, irritates the kidneys, disrupts adrenal function, depresses immunity, and agitates the nervous system. Elderly individuals frequently develop mental impairment as a result of excessive sugar intake. Parkinsonism, Alzheimer's disease, chronic depression, psychotic behavior, and senility have all been correlated with sugar overload. The fact is sugar consumption plays a greater role in the cause of these diseases than the substances typically associated with their genesis such as aluminum, iron, lead, pesticides, etc. A number of symptoms commonly experienced by the elderly, such as poor attention span, memory loss, insomnia, anxiety, agitation, irritability, confusion, hostility, fatigue, cold extremities, pruritus, and weakness, are provoked or caused by the ingestion of refined sugar. Thus, all individuals would feel better, think more clearly, and, certainly, live longer as a result of curtailing sugar intake.

As mentioned previously the average American consumption of refined sugar is over 150 pounds per person per year. Yet, this is only the average. It means that some individuals consume 200 or perhaps 300 or even more pounds of sugar per year, while others consume less. Think about it. That's two or more ten-pound bags per month. Few people would knowingly consume that much sugar. The problem is that Americans are habituated to eating food products liberally laced with a variety of refined sugars. Sugar has been added to disguise the fact that the nutrients and naturally occurring flavors have been processed out. Plus, it makes the food addictive. Sugar consumption is a habit, albeit an addictive one, not a necessity. The body has no use for this adulterated, dangerous substance. The fact is all it can do is cause damage.

REFINED SUGAR TEST (each response worth 1 point)

Do you consume on a daily, weekly, or monthly basis:
1. Hershey's, Cadbury, or other milk chocolate bars
2. Snickers, 3-Musketeers, Mars Bars, or Milky Ways
3. Nestle's Crunch or Mr. Goodbars
4. salted nut rolls
5. Butterfingers or Baby Ruths
6. (other) candy bars
7. chocolates, Hershey's kisses, or chocolate bark
8. ketchup
9. sweet relish and/or pickles
10. corn relish
11. canned sweet corn
12. pickled beets
13. cup cakes
14. brownies
15. fudge
16. sugar-sweetened cereals
17. cured luncheon meats
18. ice cream or ice milk
19. malts or shakes
20. sherbet
21. after-dinner mints
22. non-dairy creamer
23. whipping cream (artificial or canned)
24. taffy, caramels, and/or Milk Duds
25. applesauce
26. pudding
27. canned fruit in heavy or light syrup
28. honey-roasted nuts
29. homemade salad dressings sweetened with sugar
30. jelly beans
31. Juji Fruits or similar chewy treats
32. peanut butter cups
33. Zingers, Twinkies, and/or Suzi-Qs

34. oatmeal pies
35. caramel corn
36. taffy apples
37. flavored yogurt
38. vanilla wafers
39. M&M type candies
40. canned soups
41. pretzels
42. boxed soup mixes
43. graham crackers
44. Wheat and/or Oat Thins
45. jellies and jams
46. refined honey
47. apple butter
48. commercial peanut butter
49. crescent rolls
50. marshmallows and marshmallow cream
51. Pringles style potato chips
52. bread
53. hamburger and hot-dog buns
54. caramel corn, Poppy Cock, and/or Cracker Jacks
55. hot dogs
56. ham
57. bacon and/or breakfast strips
58. turkey and/or chicken salad
59. bean dip
60. Jello and/or gelatin molds
61. pickled herring
62. sausage links and/or summer sausage
63. bean and/or potato salad
64. marinara (pasta) sauce
65. canned yams
66. pickled red cabbage
67. hash browns and/or Tater Tots
68. canned chili
69. Spaghetti-Os
70. bagels

71. Sloppy Joe mix
72. steak sauce and/or taco sauce
73. barbecue sauce and/or barbecued meats
74. commercial salad dressings (mayonnaise)
75. French, Roquefort, Western, thousand island, blue cheese, ranch, and Caesar dressings
76. pancake mixes
77. frozen or prepared waffles or pancakes
78. sno-cones and/or slushes
79. Buster Bars, Dilly Bars, fudgesicles, drumsticks, or ice cream sandwiches?
80. pudding pops
81. Bomb Pops, Mr. Freeze pops, and popsicles
82. cookies
83. gum sweetened with sugar
84. hard candies
85. doughnuts
86. pies
87. pastries
88. peanut brittle
89. fruit salad
90. pecan rolls
91. Tootsie Pops and/or other suckers
92. Tootsie Rolls
93. mousses
94. baklava or similar exotic ethnic sweets
95. chutney/bottled seasonings
96. peanut clusters
97. peppermint and/or lemon drops
98. yogurt-coated nuts/candies
99. root beer floats and/or chocolate sodas
100. chocolate covered raisins, nuts, malted milk balls, etc.
101. Whip 'n Chill type desserts

Your Score _____

1 to 18 points *Mild refined sugar toxicity:* While this level of intake is listed as mild, it is still significant. It would be preferable to satisfy the desire for sweets with fresh fruits, pure raw honey, sweet vegetables, or juices. These at least contain some valuable nutrients. Be sure to take a natural-source thiamine-niacin supplement, such as Nutri-Sense, three heaping tablespoons daily. This will aid in the effort to break the sugar habit by reducing cravings. Multiple spice extracts are the most potent of all, that is for reducing sugar cravings and balancing blood sugar. Take Oregulin multiple spice oil extract, one capsule with meals. This usually produces rapid results, halting all uncontrollable sugar cravings. Fortified royal jelly (e.g. Royal Kick) is also a sugar antagonist: take two capsules daily in the morning. Not all royal jelly is the same. The Royal Kick is far more effective than the commercial type.

19 to 34 points *Moderate refined sugar toxicity:* If you suffer from fatigue, irritability, PMS, headaches, allergies, sinus problems, memory loss, irregular heartbeat, frequent colds/flu, fungal infections, itchy skin, sleep disorders, mood swings, and/or depression, sugar is the likely culprit. Refined sugar is addictive. Resolve the sugar addiction immediately before further tissue damage occurs. To aid you in this battle take a natural-source thiamine-niacin supplement, such as Nutri-Sense, three heaping tablespoons twice daily. Thiamine and niacin required to process/digest sugar and help reduce sugar cravings. Take also megadoses of tyrosine (2 grams), co-enzyme Q-10 (100 mg), and pantothenic acid (2 grams); all these nutrients boost the adrenal glands' anti-sugar response. Yet, multiple spice extracts are the most potent of all, that is for reducing sugar cravings and balancing blood sugar. Take Oregulin, one or two capsules with meals. This usually produces rapid results, halting all uncontrollable sugar cravings. To regenerate these glands take unprocessed royal jelly, i.e., Royal Kick, 4 to 6 caps every morning. Also, to help prevent sugar cravings use the sublingual form of royal jelly, i.e. Royal Oil, a squirt under the tongue as needed. Chromium also helps reverse the toxicity: take 200 or more micrograms daily.

35 to 65 points *Severe refined sugar toxicity:* You are con-suming refined sugar by the handful each day. Curtail this excessive sugar intake immediately. Follow the previously mentioned advice and take 200 to 300 mcg of chromium several times daily. Additionally, take magnesium (1 gram), potassium (300 mg), selenium (300 mcg), manganese (15 mg), and silica (500 mg), since sugar induces deficiencies of all of these nutrients. Take also megadoses of pantothenic acid, 1500 mg three or four times daily. Yet, multiple spice extracts are the most potent of all, that is for reducing sugar cravings and balancing blood sugar. Take Oregulin as the preferred and most potent supplement, two or more capsules with meals (for those who wish not to take gelatin capsules it is available as liquid drops). This usually produces rapid results, halting all uncontrollable sugar cravings. Do whatever it takes to lick the sugar habit. The adrenal glands are greatly damaged by this degree of sugar intake. To regenerate them take Royal Kick, 6 caps every morning. Usually, significant results are noticed within a month. To regenerate these glands take unprocessed royal jelly, i.e., Royal Kick, 4 caps every morning. Also, to help prevent sugar cravings use the sublingual form of royal jelly, i.e. Royal Oil, a squirt under the tongue as needed.

66 and above *Extreme refined sugar toxicity:* You are con-suming refined sugar by the bowlful each day (or each week). As a result your internal organs literally are becoming corroded. The greatest damage is being inflicted upon the liver, colon, pancreas, adrenal glands, thyroid gland, and pituitary gland. Stop this destructive sugar addiction immediately. Take a natural-source niacin-thiamine supplement, that is Nutri-Sense, three heaping tablespoons twice daily. Also, take chromium, 400 mcg twice daily as well as megadoses of pantothenic acid, 2000 mg three times daily. Selenium and zinc help reverse sugar toxicity: on a daily basis take 400 mcg and 75 mg respectively. In order to reverse the toxicity the thyroid function may need to be balanced: take ThyroNorm, three capsules twice daily. Yet, multiple spice extracts are the most potent of all, that is for reducing sugar cravings and balancing blood sugar. Take Oregulin as the preferred and most potent supplement, two or more capsules with meals (for those who wish not to take gelatin capsules it is available as liquid drops). To regenerate these glands take unprocessed royal jelly, i.e., Royal Kick, 4 caps every morning and also 4 at noon. Also, to help prevent sugar cravings use the sublingual form of royal jelly, i.e. Royal Oil, a squirt under the tongue as needed.

After breaking the sugar habit remain on the supplements for at least 90 days. Then, as a maintenance reduce the dosage by 50% as a maintenance.

Refined Sugar in Beverages

Here is an astounding statistic: Americans consume a greater volume of fluid as soft drinks than water. If beer were included as a soft drink (it is more hard than soft), water would be a major loser.

Soft drinks are a primary source of sugar in the American diet. In fact, these drinks constitute fully 25% of all sugar consumption. The sugar in these drinks is readily disguised by a variety of coloring agents (including caramel) if not subtly by the colorful graphics of the soft drink containers. It is bizarre that people drink soft drinks without considering that all they are getting nutritionally is pure sugar. These same individuals might think twice about drinking the homemade equivalent of a typical cola: seven to eight teaspoons of white sugar stirred into a twelve ounce glass of carbonated water. The fact is virtually no one would willingly drink such a concoction. Yet, in the disguised form billions of people do so every day. However, it is not just soft drinks that are major sources of "drinkable" sugar. There are literally hundreds of other drinks containing it, many of which are listed as follows:

REFINED SUGAR IN BEVERAGES TEST
(each response worth 1 point)

Do you consume on a daily or weekly basis:

1. Kool Aid
2. colas (including Dr. Pepper)
3. Hi-C and/or fruit punch
4. grape, lemon, lime, or orange juice drink
5. chocolate milk
6. hot chocolate (or hot cocoa)
7. coffee or tea with sugar
8. coffee or tea with coffee creamer
9. Ovaltine, PDQ, or Nestle's Quick
10. instant breakfast
11. Slim-Fast or similar weight loss drinks
12. lemonade
13. malted milk
14. malts and shakes
15. ice cream sodas
16. ice slushes
17. sweetened ice tea
18. "health drinks" sweetened with grape sugar, apple juice, or corn syrup
19. refined apple juice
20. peach, pear, apricot, or guava nectar
21. cranberry juice cocktail
22. liqueurs
23. mixed drinks containing added sugar

24. Gatorade and/or similar athletic drinks
25. Ensure and/or similar supplemental drinks
26. Tang
27. 7-Up, Sprite, or Mountain Dew
28. root beer
29. fruit flavored sodas (Orange Crush, grape soda, etc.)
30. Do you drink 2 or more cans/bottles of pop every day? (If so, add 3 additional points to your total)

Your Score _____

---

1 to 5 points   *Mild sugary drink toxicity*
6 to 12 points   *Moderate sugary drink toxicity*
13 to 19 points   *Severe sugary drink toxicity*
20 and above   *Extreme sugary drink toxicity*

For all categories the treatment is the same; stop consuming drinks containing sugar, corn syrup, caffeine, and food dyes. Drink instead beverages that are health-enhancing such as pure fruit and vegetable juices, unsweetened protein shakes (such as Nutri-Sense mixed with fruit and yogurt), and water. Individuals who score on the high end of the severe or extreme category have an increased risk for certain illnesses, notably low blood sugar, diabetes, tooth decay, pyorrhea, anxiety, depression, lupus, PMS, endometriosis, and heart disease. Additionally, excessive intake of sugar greatly impairs the immune response, predisposing individuals to a wide range of infectious conditions, including colds, flu, pneumonia, bronchitis, ear infections, and, particularly, yeast infections. This is largely because sugar destroys selenium, zinc, vitamin C, pantothenic acid, and pyridoxine, all of which are necessary for maintenance of normal immunity. The adrenal glands are significantly damaged by refined sugar. To reverse this damage take crude royal jelly, i.e., Royal Kick, 4 to 6 caps every morning.

Food Dyes

Food processors are convinced that foods must be adulterated with artificial colors in order to make them appear more appetizing. Thus, they add all manner of food colorings to enhance visual appeal and stimulate purchasing. No consideration is given by the food processors regarding the food value or potential toxicity of these dyes. Rather, the only concern is "what will sell". Thus, thousands of foods contain synthetic dyes made from coal tar and petrochemical residues, these dyes being descriptively known as artificial colors.

I observed an interesting event illustrating the effects of food dyes on living tissues. I was in the wilderness—fishing in Canada. One of our party was far from nutritionally oriented; he brought along a couple of quarts of Gatorade. This drink consists largely of refined sugar and food dyes. We caught and cleaned fish from the pristine waters of the Canadian wilderness—pure white fillets of walleyed pike. The fish were placed in the refrigerator with the intent of preparing them later for supper. When I removed them, the flesh of the fish had turned pink—the Gatorade, since it was placed on its side in the small refrigerator, had leaked into the fish container. The red dye had leached into the fish, essentially "pickling them" irreparably, and no amount of washing could salvage them. I explained to my companion that this was precisely what was happening to his internal organs when he consumed Gatorade or similar drinks laced with food dyes.

The FDA keeps tabs on food dyes by issuing numbers for each of them. You can tell if a food dye is synthetic and, therefore, toxic in two ways: if the label lists the terminology "artificial color(s)" or if it is listed as a numbered dye such as FD&C #5. All these dyes are documented carcinogens. My philosophy is no level is safe. Carefully read all labels and avoid foods containing artificial dyes. Certainly, do not add food dyes to your foods. It is possible to have a happy Easter without coating eggs with toxic food dyes.

FOOD DYE TEST (each response worth 1 point)

Do you consume on a daily, weekly, or monthly basis:

1. pickles
2. relish
3. dinner rolls (some)
4. popsicles
5. Kool-Aid
6. gelatin
7. hard candies
8. chewing gum (or bubble gum)
9. Gatorade and similar artificially colored sports drinks
10. sno-cones and slushes
11. fruit drinks and/or punch
12. puddings
13. pie fillings
14. frostings
15. artificial cheese and processed sliced cheeses
16. canned fruit
17. colored cereals
18. marshmallows (colored or white)
19. sherbet
20. Mountain Dew
21. apple and cherry turnovers
22. wine coolers
23. commercial multiple vitamins
24. coated or colored drugs
25. red, orange, yellow, blue, or green colored candies
26. birthday and/or layer cakes
27. fruit, upside down, and tea cakes
28. imitation cheese
29. maraschino cherries and/or crab apples
30. frozen pizzas
31. microwave popcorn
32. Trix, Lucky Charms, Fruit Loops, and similar colored cereals

33. thousand island dressing
34. ice cream (especially fruit-flavored)
35. canned frosting
36. orange, yellow, or green colored pop
37. Cool Whip or similar imitation whipped toppings
38. grape or orange drink (including Hi-C)
39. Pop Tarts
40. pudding pops
41. margarine
42. crescent rolls (and also some hotdog/hamburger buns)
43. doughnuts
44. sweet rolls
45. commercial cheese cake

Your Score ____

---

1 to 8 points *Mild food dye toxicity:* Even in minute quantities food dyes are toxic. These chemicals are proven carcinogens. Avoid them as you would avoid the plague. Do not feed your children food dye-contaminated foods. Such dyes are a primary cause of certain diseases, notably attention deficit disorder, learning disabilities, asthma, and migraine headaches.

9 to 18 points *Moderate food dye toxicity:* You are consuming excessive amounts of processed foods contaminated with food dyes. Change your diet by eating wholesome, unprocessed foods instead of devitalized, chemically poisoned foods. To neutralize food dye toxicity, take Oregacyn, one capsule twice daily.

19 to 28 points *Severe food dye toxicity:* At this level of intake a variety of symptoms are likely to occur, including depression, headaches, agitation, joint pain, fatigue, sinus problems, cold/flu, and irritability. In children food dyes may cause or provoke a variety of mental illnesses such as attention deficit disorder, behavioral defects, delayed learning, depression, autism, and even seizures. They are also related to the cause of asthma, sinusitis, and bronchitis.

Asthmatics are particularly vulnerable to the toxic effects of food dyes and may exhibit severe allergic reactions. In fact, thousands of fatal and near fatal reactions have resulted from the ingestion of food dyes. The main culprit is Yellow Dye #5. Also known as tartrazine, this coal tar derivative is the asthmatic's processed food nightmare. The chemical belongs to the aspirin family. Thus, aspirin-sensitive asthmatics, of which there are millions, are exceptionally sensitive to it. Asthmatics must scrutinize the labels of all processed foods for such terms as food dyes, artificial colorings, artificial flavorings, tartrazine, and Yellow Dye #5. To strengthen the adrenal glands and combat allergic reactions take crude fortified royal jelly, i.e. Royal Kick, 4 capsules daily. Also, to detoxify the poisonous effects of these dyes take Gene's greens, 2 dropperfuls twice daily and take Oregacyn, 1-2 capsules twice daily.

29 and above *Extreme food dye toxicity:* Warning—the consumption of large amounts of food dyes over prolonged periods increases the risks for a variety of cancers. Follow the previously mentioned advice, being sure to carefully eliminate all dietary sources of these carcinogens. Individuals suffering from chronic disease who registered in the extreme category will invariably notice an improvement after eliminating dietary sources of synthetic dyes.

It is essential that you regard this advice seriously and alter your diet immediately. If you are an asthmatic, removing food dyes from the diet may be a matter of life and death. To strengthen the adrenal glands in order to reverse toxicity take crude fortified royal jelly, i.e. Royal Kick, 6 capsules daily. Also, to detoxify the poisonous effects of these dyes take Gene's greens, 3 droppers full twice daily and take Oregacyn, 2 capsules twice daily.

MSG

MSG, or monosodium glutamate, is a synthetic chemical which is commonly added to processed foods. It is described on some food labels as a "flavor enhancer". It is devoid of nutritional value. In fact, even in relatively small quantities it is toxic. The point is this is a completely synthetic substance, which offers no benefits to the body.

Dr. George Schwartz's book, *In Bad Taste: The MSG Syndrome*, classifies MSG as a drug-like substance. Further, he claims that "MSG is a poison...," which would not be surprising, since drugs produce their actions by poisoning cellular functions. To illustrate the widespread occurrence of MSG in foods, Dr. Schwartz notes that MSG is found in *"most of the food* prepared by major fast-food chains (italics mine)." Moreover, he notes that as many as 20 million Americans, or nearly one-tenth of the population, are known MSG reactors. He proposes that in all probability this figure could be tripled to include those who are unknowingly sensitive to it. This latter figure is supported by laboratory data. Studies on MSG toxicity describe a consistent picture; nearly one-third of animals and humans tested reacted negatively in some fashion after ingesting MSG. What's more, certain subjects developed intense and potentially dangerous symptoms. The researchers concluded that in highly sensitive individuals permanent disability may result from toxic MSG reactions.

MSG is truly a hidden food additive. Usually, it can't be seen, touched, smelled, or even tasted. To make matters worse it is often disguised on food labels under names besides MSG. Schwartz notes that the term MSG is less commonly found on food labels than the toxin's disguised names: hydrolyzed vegetable protein, autolyzed yeast, modified food starch, and "natural" flavors. Thousands of processed foods have these terms listed on their labels, and all are taboo for those who are MSG-sensitive, rather, for anyone who wishes to have exceptional health.

MSG TEST (each response worth one point)

Do you consume:
1. fish sticks or patties
2. tortilla chips
3. potato chips
4. Cheetos or cheese puffs
5. soy sauce
6. canned stew
7. processed cheese
8. Planters dry roasted nuts (other brands also may contain MSG)
9. croutons and bread crumbs
10. canned tuna (Chicken of the Sea, Geisha, Bumble Bee, or S&W)
11. canned chunky beef, chicken, or turkey
12. canned chicken, ham, turkey, or beef spread
13. canned Chinese foods
14. canned ravioli, Beefaroni, or spaghetti and meatballs
15. pizza (especially frozen types)
16. egg rolls
17. breaded chicken (i.e. fried chicken, chicken nuggets, etc.)
18. TV dinners
19. breaded shrimp, clams, and/or scallops
20. submarine sandwiches
21. pepperoni
22. hot dogs and/or corn dogs
23. bologna and/or salami
24. pastrami
25. tenderloins
26. breakfast strips
27. egg substitutes
28. baked beans
29. creamed vegetables

30. scalloped and/or au gratin potatoes
31. tomato sauce (some)
32. chili
33. prepared sliced turkey, beef, or chicken (deli-style)
34. Sloppy Joe mix
35. pudding
36. taco sauce
37. ketchup
38. tartar sauce (some)
39. mayonnaise
40. thousand island dressing
41. French, ranch, or Caesar dressing
42. chicken-fried, Salisbury, or Swiss steak
43. beef Stroganoff
44. artificial ice cream
45. frozen waffles
46. cream soups
47. broth soups and/or canned soup broth
48. steaks, chops, or poultry seasoned with Accent or Lawry's seasoning
49. Oriental restaurant food
50. boxed soup mixes
51. chunky soups
52. doughnuts, sweet rolls, and/or cupcakes
53. fruit pies
54. cup cakes
55. bean dip
56. cheese dip (some)
57. peanut butter cookies (some)
58. flavored yogurt (some)

Your Score _____

---

1 to 10 points Mild MSG toxicity: If you are an MSG reactor, even tiny amounts must be avoided. This is particularly true if you suffer from allergy-induced illnesses such as arthritis, hyperactivity, attention deficit disorder, asthma, hives, obesity, or migraines.

11 to 22 points Moderate MSG toxicity: You are consuming a significant amount of MSG on a daily or weekly basis. It is likely that the MSG is accumulating in your tissues and causing toxicity. This can result in a variety of mental symptoms and may ultimately contribute to the cause of certain diseases. Curtail the consumption of MSG and MSG-tainted foods. The following nutrients may be useful in reducing MSG toxicity:

- vitamin C - 1,000 mg twice daily
- vitamin E - 1200 I.U. daily
- selenium - 400 mcg daily
- beta carotene - 25,000 I.U. daily
- fat-soluble thiamine - 200 mg daily
- B-complex - 1 tablet twice daily
- oil of wild oregano (Oreganol) - 3 to 5 drops twice daily

23 to 41 points *Severe MSG toxicity:* You are consuming large amounts of MSG on a daily basis. Migraine headaches, flu-like symptoms, sinusitis, memory loss, depression, agitation, and anxiety are common MSG-induced syndromes. The consumption of this compound is probably responsible for many of your ailments. In all likelihood you are addicted to MSG, and the reactions it causes in your body may be turning you into a nervous wreck. Go cold turkey and remove all dietary sources of MSG. Take the following nutritional supplements to aid in preventing withdrawal symptoms and to heal any toxic damage that may have developed within the nervous system:

- vitamin C - 1,000 mg three times daily
- vitamin E - 800 I.U. daily

- selenium - 300 mcg twice daily
- natural-source niacin and thiamine (i.e. Nutri-Sense) – 3 teaspoons daily
- tyrosine - 1 gram twice daily
- B-complex - 1 tablet three times daily
- magnesium - 400 mg twice daily
- Oregacyn Mind/Memory – 2 caps twice daily
- B-6 - 50 mg daily
- Essence of orange blossom (helps regenerate damaged brain waves) - 2 tablespoons in hot water daily
- oil of wild oregano (Oreganol) - 5 drops twice daily

42 and above Extreme MSG toxicity: Warning—neurological damage may occur as a result of prolonged consumption of large amounts of MSG. At this level of intake MSG-induced imbalances in brain chemistry are virtually assured. Severe depression, agitation, and even suicidal ideation may result. To help reverse MSG-induced damage and neurological imbalances, as well as to aid in curing the addiction, take the following brain chemistry enhancing agents:

- tyrosine - 1 gram twice daily
- natural-source niacin and thiamine (i.e. Nutri-Sense) – three heaping tablespoons twice daily
- B-complex - 2 tablets three times daily
- B-6 - 50 mg twice daily
- folic acid - 5 mg twice daily
- magnesium - 400 mg twice daily
- calcium - 500 mg twice daily
- fat-soluble thiamine - 200 mg three times daily
- Essence of orange blossom (helps regenerate damaged brain mechanisms) - 2 to 4 tablespoons in hot water daily
- Oregacyn Mind/Memory formula – 2 caps twice daily

In addition, take the following antioxidants in order to heal the nervous system damage/toxicity:

- natural-source vitamin C (i.e. Flavin-C) – 3 caps twice daily
- vitamin E - 800 I.U. daily
- selenium - 250 mcg twice daily
- glutathione - 200 mg twice daily
- essential fatty acids - 9 capsules daily
- Oreganol (oil of wild oregano) - 5 to 10 drops twice daily

There is a highly effective way to neutralize MSG reactions: oil of wild oregano, that is the Oreganol. Simply take a few drops under the tongue at the beginning of any reaction and repeat until symptoms dissipate.

Sulfites

Sulfites are a class of chemicals derived from the gaseous compound sulfur dioxide. The toxicity of sulfur dioxide is well known. This is the compound responsible for acid rain.

Sulfites and sulfur dioxide are added to foods in order to preserve their appearance. Sulfites offer no nutritional value and, in fact, destroy nutrients, notably vitamin C, vitamin A, vitamin B, vitamin B-12, riboflavin, and molybdenum. Asthmatics are particularly vulnerable to reacting to the toxicity of sulfites, and several deaths have occurred as a result of sulfite allergy.

Dozens of symptoms result from sulfite reactions. These symptoms include rashes (particularly hives), sinus congestion or runny nose, sinus pressure, headaches, achiness, cold sweats, diarrhea, joint pain, chest pain, shortness of breath, swelling of the face, throat, tongue, or lips, and sudden bouts of fatigue. Sulfites are unfit for human consumption.

SULFITES TEST (each response worth 1 point)

Do you consume:

1. cole slaw
2. dried fruits
3. white and brown sugar
4. potato salad
5. pies
6. hard candy
7. gelatin (Jello)
8. fruit drinks
9. fruit salad (fresh, frozen, or canned)
10. frozen vegetables
11. guacamole
12. tortilla chips
13. canned soups
14. deli fruit or salads
15. fruit toppings and fillings
16. jams and jellies
17. pancake mixes
18. pancake syrup
19. cornstarch
20. instant tea
21. hard liquor
22. breakfast drinks
23. gravies and sauces
24. salad dressings
25. TV dinners
26. French fries, Tater Tots, or American fries
27. hash browns
28. horseradish (some)
29. frozen fruit (some)
30. sauerkraut
31. scalloped or au gratin potatoes

32. instant mashed potatoes
33. soy sauce (some)
34. vinegar (most)
35. fruit pies
36. wine and wine coolers
37. restaurant foods cooked in wine

Your Score _____

---

1 to 7 points *Mild sulfite toxicity:* Even at this low level of intake highly sensitive individuals might exhibit toxicity. Usually, such individuals have a history of allergy manifested by asthmatic attacks, allergic rashes, hives, sinus problems, and/or migraine headaches. Individuals who exhibit sensitivity must avoid all dietary sources of sulfites.

8 to 19 points *Moderate sulfite toxicity:* Sulfites are poisonous and, once ingested, are converted to the highly toxic gas, sulfur dioxide. Sulfites and their metabolites suppress immunity and provoke allergic reactions. Curtail the consumption of all food containing sulfites and take the following nutrients in order to detoxify the residues of this poison:

- vitamin B-12 - 500 mcg daily
- folic acid - 1 mg daily
- natural vitamin C plus bioflavonoids (e.g. Flavin-C) - 3 caps twice daily
- molybdenum - 100 mcg twice daily
- oil of wild Oreganol - five drops twice daily

Note: the Oreganol will neutralize acute sulfite reactions.

20 to 28 points *Severe sulfite toxicity:* Warning—serious injury and/or death may occur in highly sensitive individuals as a result of the consumption of large amounts of sulfites. Allergic reactions to sulfites include hives, rashes, sinus disturbances, headaches, shortness of breath, and sore throats. Avoid all dietary sources of sulfites and take the following supplements:

- vitamin B-12 - 1,000 mcg daily
- folic acid - 2 mg twice daily
- natural vitamin C plus bioflavonoids (e.g. Flavin-C) - 3 caps twice daily
- molybdenum - 50 mcg three times daily
- selenium - 200 mcg twice daily
- methyl sulfonyl methane (MSM) - 150 mg twice daily
- oil of wild Oreganol - ten drops twice daily

29 and above *Extreme sulfite toxicity:* You are consuming massive amounts of the highly oxidative sulfites on a daily basis. If you have a significant history of allergy and/or asthma, your life may be at risk. Sulfite-induced asthmatic attacks, throat edema, and shock are serious reactions; dozens of deaths have resulted from such toxic insults. Immediately curtail the intake of all dietary sources of sulfites. Always ask the preparers/servers at restaurants if sulfites are added to the food. In addition, take the following sulfite antagonists and detoxifying agents:

- vitamin B-12 - 1,000 mcg three times daily
- folic acid - 2 mg three times daily
- natural vitamin C (e.g. Flavin-C) - 3 caps three times daily
- vitamin A - 25,000 I.U. twice daily
- molybdenum - 200 mcg three times daily
- organic selenium - 200 mcg twice daily
- N-acetyl cysteine - 100 mg twice daily
- oil of wild Oreganol - 10 to 20 drops twice daily (or if using gelcaps, 2 twice daily)

Nitrated Meats

Nitrates are added to meats as preservatives, primarily to prevent microbial growth. However, they also are utilized to improve visual appeal, since they turn the meat a brighter color, giving it a reddish tint. Excessive dietary intake of nitrates is linked to heart disease, diabetes, stroke, and cancer.

The cancer-causing effects of nitrates have been thoroughly investigated. When nitrates or nitrites are ingested, they are converted in the stomach and intestines to compounds of even greater toxicity called *nitrosamines*. The toxicity of nitrosamines is so profound that they are regarded as one of the most potent of all known carcinogens. Nitrosamines damage the lining of the stomach and intestines by destroying cellular genetic material. Chronic consumption of nitrates with subsequent formation into nitrosamines significantly increases the risks for stomach, intestinal, esophageal, bladder, and liver cancer.

The transformation of nitrates to nitrosamines is blocked by certain foods, vitamins, and minerals. Researchers discovered that nitrosamine formation within the intestines can be prevented, that is if the diet is rich in vitamin C. Other nutrients which inactivate nitrosamines and/or prevent their formation include beta carotene, glutathione, selenium, bioflavonoids, riboflavin, and vitamin E. Aged garlic extract is even more powerful than these nutrients. Recent research conducted in Asia determined that garlic extract (Kyolic was the brand used) was ten times more effective than vitamin C in inactivating nitrosamines. Other pungent foods and spices are equally effective, notably wild oregano blends, that is Oreganol, as well as oils of cumin and rosemary. The Oreganol aggressively neutralizes nitrosamine poisoning.

Cigarette smoke is another major source of nitrosamines. Every puff initiates a chain reaction leading to nitrosamine formation within the tissues, particularly the lungs, liver, and digestive tract. In fact, according to the internationally renowned cancer researcher Kedar Prasad, author of *Vitamins*

Against Cancer, cigarette smoke is the number one environmental source of nitrosamines. This largely accounts for the powerful cancer-causing actions of tobacco smoke. Here, the wild oregano is highly effective. It halts both the symptoms of smoke toxicity, such as lung and sinus disorders, while neutralizing nitrosamine formation. The fact is certain smokers have found the oil invaluable in helping to curb or even eliminate the habit. The key appears to be frequent use such as a few drops under the tongue at the moment of any craving.

Tap water is an additional significant source of nitrates. The major source of nitrates in water is agricultural run-off of nitrogenous fertilizers and animal wastes. When ingested these nitrates can also be converted to nitrosamines.

NITRATED MEATS TEST (each response worth 1 point)

Do you consume:

1. pork and beans
2. ham
3. salami and/or summer sausage
4. bologna
5. head cheese and/or pickled pigs feet
6. bacon and/or breakfast strips
7. corned beef and/or corned beef hash
8. pastrami
9. hot dogs and/or corn dogs
10. smoked turkey breast
11. Spam
12. sausage
13. turkey salami, bologna, or ham
14. beef jerky
15. chipped beef
16. bratwurst
17. liverwurst
18. pepperoni and/or Canadian bacon

19. Do you eat smoked fish (including lox)?
20. Do you eat fresh fruits and vegetables only rarely?
21. Do you live in an area of heavy air pollution?
22. Do you smoke cigarettes on a daily basis? (Note: if you smoked 2 packs or more for longer than five years, add an additional 4 points)
23. Are you exposed to passive smoke on a daily basis?
24. Do you smoke pipes or cigars?
25. Do you use chewing tobacco?
26. Do you drink tap water derived from water tables in an area of heavy agriculture?

Your Score _____

---

1 to 6 points *Mild nitrate toxicity:* Nitrosamines are potent carcinogens. Thus, no amount of dietary intake of nitrates can be deemed safe. Since nitrates and particularly nitrites are readily converted to nitrosamines, the consumption of nitrated meats should be restricted or preferably curtailed. Be sure to take oil of wild oregano (i.e. Oreganol) as well as extra amounts of natural vitamin C, for instance, Flavin-C, 2 caps twice daily. Natural vitamin C works in the body in a more efficient way than synthetic. Plus, it is better retained by the cells. The regular intake of natural vitamin C, both in supplements and as food extracts, will help clear the noxious nitrates out of the system. Drink a large glass of fresh citrus juice daily.

7 to 12 points *Moderate nitrate toxicity:* At this level of intake the risks for cancer and heart disease rise significantly. Eliminate all dietary sources of nitrates, including smoked foods. Avoid barbecued meats. Protect yourself from unavoidable secondhand smoke and pollution by taking large doses of antioxidants, particularly vitamin E, beta carotene, vitamin A, vitamin C, selenium, and glutathione. Take also Oregacyn multi-spice antioxidant caps, 2 caps twice daily. The regular intake of natural vitamin C, both in supplements and as food extracts, will help clear the noxious nitrates from the system. Drink a large glass of fresh citrus juice daily.

13 to 18 points *Severe nitrate toxicity:* Warning—the amount of nitrates you are consuming greatly increases your risks for heart disease and cancer. Stop the intake of all nitrated and smoked meats. If you are a smoker, quit immediately. If you are exposed to significant amounts of second hand smoke, do whatever is necessary to protect yourself, e.g. make your spouse smoke outside the house, etc. Use the oil of oregano to help you quit or to protect you from second-hand smoke. The consumption of large doses of antioxidants and other nutrients which prevent or reverse nitrate-induced toxicity will help stimulate the healing of damaged tissues. Take the following nutrients on a daily basis for at least two months:

- organic selenium - 600 mcg
- beta carotene - 100,000 I.U.
- natural vitamin C (e.g. Flavin-C) - 4 caps twice daily
- vitamin B - 1600 I.U.
- glutathione - 300 mg
- zinc - 50mg
- pantothenic acid - 2,000 mg
- vitamin B-6 - 50 mg
- folic acid - 5 mg
- Oregacyn multiple spice extract - 3 capsules twice daily
- Oreganol oil of wild oregano - 10 drops twice daily

Note: wild oregano is the most potent agent for neutralizing nitrate and nitrite toxicity. The regular intake of natural vitamin C, both in supplements and as food extracts, will help clear the noxious nitrates from the system. Drink a large glass of fresh citrus juice daily.

19 and above *Extreme nitrate toxicity*: You are consuming nitrates and nitrites by the teaspoonful. Nitrosamine formation is assuredly occurring in your internal organs. The risk for developing life-threatening diseases, particularly cancer, heart disease, and diabetes, is exceedingly high. If you are a migraine headache, arthritis, or asthma sufferer, it is likely that dietary nitrates are contributing to the cause. If you are a smoker, your life is at risk unless you quit immediately. Stop consuming nitrated meats and/or other sources of nitrates, before it is too late. Follow the supplemental program listed previously; however, increase the dosage of glutathione to 500 mg and vitamin E to 1200 I.U. The regular intake of natural vitamin C, both in supplements and as food extracts, will help clear the noxious nitrates out of the system. Natural vitamin C is more readily tolerated than the synthetic. As a natural source take Flavin-C, 4 to 6 caps twice daily. Also, drink two large glasses of fresh citrus juice daily. Take the Oreganol, 10 drops twice daily, and if a smoker, use it at the moment of any craving. It may also be used to neutralize the toxicity of chewing tobacco.

Caffeine and Caffeine-Like Substance

Caffeine can be descriptively called the "nervousness" food additive. It is one of the most powerful of all addictive substances, and millions of Americans are knowingly or unknowingly habituated. However, caffeine addicts don't take this substance simply to get wound up. Rather, they consume it because it gives them a jolt of energy, albeit temporary. Since the energy they receive is artificial, caffeine addicts continually consume it to maintain the sensation of nervous energy.

Caffeine is technically listed as a drug. The fact is it is an ingredient in dozens of over-the-counter as well as prescription medications. Yet, it is freely added to foods in amounts which produce drug-like effects.

This test evaluates the consumption of food/beverage sources of caffeine, as well as caffeine-like substances, the latter being found primarily in cocoa- and vanilla-flavored foods. Both cocoa and vanilla beans contain nervous system stimulants from the same chemical family as caffeine. These stimulants are known collectively as *methylxanthines.*

Caffeine is a neurotoxin. If consumed continually, it readily accumulates within the tissues, since it takes approximately eight hours to fully metabolize. What's more, it tends to preferentially accumulate within the tissues of the nervous system: the brain, spinal cord, and peripheral nerves. Thus, with repeated daily doses, it is possible to develop caffeine toxicity. This is especially true for those suffering from liver or kidney disease, since these organs are involved in the excretion and detoxification of this substance. In other words, if the function of these organs is impaired, toxic amounts of caffeine rapidly accumulate in the tissues.

CAFFEINE TEST (each response worth 1 point)

Do you consume on a daily or weekly basis:

1. caffeinated coffee
2. iced tea
3. black or green tea
4. herbal teas containing black tea
5. colas containing caffeine
6. Mountain Dew
7. chocolates or chocolate-coated candy bars
8. chocolate milk
9. cookies containing chocolate chips
10. chocolate malts, shakes, and/or sodas
11. chocolate covered ice cream bars
12. coffee flavored candy and/or ice cream
13. cookies flavored with cocoa or vanilla bean extract

14. chocolate or vanilla flavored cake
15. ice cream flavored with cocoa or vanilla bean extract
16. candy bars containing vanilla bean extract
17. chocolate or vanilla pudding
18. chocolate mousse or Whip 'n Chill
19. brownies or fudge
20. almond bark
21. cappuccino
22. hot chocolate
23. Dr. Pepper
24. Are you currently taking theophylline (asthma medication)?
25. Do you have a history of endometriosis and/or fibrocystic breast disease?
26. Do you consume drugs which contain caffeine (e.g. Excedrin, Caffergot, etc.)?
27. Do you have a history of kidney and/or liver disease?
28. Do your hands tremble after consuming caffeinated substances?
29. Do you become nervous, moody, and/or agitated after consuming caffeinated substances?
30. Do you develop a headache, or do you become irritable if you fail to get your caffeine fix?
31. Do you binge on and/or crave chocolate (for heavy chocolate eaters add an additional 4 points)?
32. Do you drink 6 or more cups of coffee per day? (if so, add an additional 4 points to your final score)?

Your Score _____

1 to 6 points *Mild Caffeine Toxicity:* For some individuals caffeine is toxic in any amount. This may be partially the result of an allergy-like sensitivity to the substance. If you are caffeine-sensitive or if you have a history of PMS, endometriosis, migraine headaches, ulcerative colitis, or fibrocystic breast disease, avoid even small amounts of caffeine and caffeine-like substances.

7 to 15 points *Moderate Caffeine Toxicity:* You are consuming excessive amounts of caffeine and caffeine-like substances on a daily or weekly basis. As a result, a variety of symptoms are probably occurring, including insomnia, agitation, nervousness, mood swings, breast tenderness, PMS, migraines, colitis, tremors, and headaches. If you have symptoms of caffeine-induced illness, curtail the consumption of all dietary sources of caffeine, cocoa, and vanilla bean. In addition, take the following supplements in order to detoxify the residual caffeine:

- pantothenic acid - 1,000 mg twice daily
- vitamin C - 500 mg twice daily
- selenium - 200 mcg twice daily
- tyrosine - 500 mg twice daily
- choline - 500 mg twice daily
- vitamin B-6 - 25 mg twice daily
- fortified royal jelly - 4 caps twice daily

16 to 23 points *Severe Caffeine Toxicity:* The caffeine you are consuming is causing toxicity within your nervous system. Immediately stop the intake of dietary sources of caffeine. However, due to the risk of withdrawal reactions, go cold turkey only after beginning the following nutritional supplement program:

- pantothenic acid - 1,000 mg twice daily
- vitamin C - 1,000 mg twice daily
- folic acid - 1 mg twice daily
- B-complex - 1 tab twice daily
- tyrosine - 1,000 mg twice daily
- vitamin B-6 - 50 mg twice daily
- choline - 500 mg twice daily
- fortified royal jelly - 4 caps three times daily

270 Nutrition Tests for Better Health

24 and above *Extreme Caffeine Toxicity:* Warning—caffeine and/or coffee, if consumed in massive amounts, may cause genetic damage. Studies document that heavy coffee consumption results in damage to genetic material, which has been determined by detecting the existence of abnormal chromosomes in the urine. In addition, the risk for pancreatic cancer is significantly increased for those who consume in excess of five cups of coffee per day. Curtail the excessive caffeine/coffee consumption immediately. Be aware of the side effects of going cold turkey: depression, agitation, anxiety, nervousness, shaking/tremors, anger, frustration, insomnia, digestive disturbances, constipation, fatigue, and headaches. To help control or minimize these symptoms initiate the following nutritional supplement program prior to discontinuing the caffeine:

- folic acid - 1 mg three times daily
- B-complex - 1 tab three times daily
- ThyroNorm - 2 to 3 caps three times daily
- Oreganol oil of wild oregano - 5 drops twice daily
- fortified royal jelly - 4 caps three times daily
- fat-soluble thiamine - 300 mg twice daily
- selenium - 300 mcg twice daily

Note: the fortified royal jelly, that is the Royal Kick, is the most crucial of all caffeine-detoxification substances. This is because it boosts adrenal function, helping prevent withdrawal. It may be taken frequently to prevent nervousness, agitation, and/or headache. Because Royal Kick is a high grade supplement, it is far superior to the commercial types. Royal Kick may not be found in stores. To order call 1-800-243-5242.

Section III
Illnesses and Syndromes

Excessive Aging

No one wants to become old. Yet, everyone must deal with this issue. While ageing is inevitable, a person can largely preserve his/her appearance as well as health. In other words, it is far from inevitable to look excessively old. Nor is it a requirement to lose teeth, develop failing eyesight, suffer hearing loss, become bald and/or gray, or shrivel up like a prune. Rather, aging can be blocked, delayed, or controlled. Thus, it is possible to retain a certain degree of vitality and vigor, as well as a youthful appearance, despite reaching old age. A "feel and act young" attitude is essential, but so is an adequate supply of the nutrients which stall the aging process. This is because aging occurs primarily from the inside out and the essential nutrients decrease the rate of aging that occurs within internal organs.

Certain nutrients have been studied extensively for their anti-aging properties. These nutrients exert their effects whether taken internally or applied externally. In fact, the combination of external and internal application of anti-aging nutrition is one of the secrets to maintaining beauty and physique well into old age. As only one example of the value of nutrients in reversing aging, researchers reported that taking vitamin C supplements on a regular basis may extend life span by as much as six years. The regular intake of natural-source vitamin C, from foods and supplements, is also life-extending. Just think what could be accomplished in aging delay if a broad spectrum of anti-aging nutrients were consumed on a regular basis.

Certain dietary factors accelerate aging. Excessive eating is one of them. The per capita caloric consumption in America is astronomically high and is nearly twice that of primitive societies. Researchers have thoroughly documented the fact that fasting or moderate food abstinence helps retard the aging process and may extend life span by as much as ten years.

The Islamic fast is notable. Here, for a month each year people abstain from food and drink for twelve hours or more every day. This complete resting of the gut stalls both aging and the onset of disease. This is because such a fast halts the oxidative damage, which accelerates aging. It also helps preserve the digestive juices, which also delays aging. Thus, the Islamic fast is the ideal type, because it causes a complete preservation of the digestive process. Plus, since it is performed regularly it aids in the stalling of the aging process. Again, in modern society overeating is the primary cause of aging. For more information on the scientific basis of the Islamic text see the book, *Science and Religion* (Knowledge House: Dr. K. Khaleel).

The skin is a barometer of how rapidly an individual is aging. Americans often marvel at how elderly individuals from non-Western societies appear young and how their skin remains beautiful. These individuals follow a diet closer to an "all-natural" one which is relatively free of the toxic substances replete in the American diet. These toxic substances may be descriptively called *aging factors*. They include refined vegetable oils, hydrogenated oils, refined sugar, inorganic iron, nitrates, synthetic food additives, caffeine, and cigarette smoke (separate exams are found within this book for each of these items).

There are a number of external as well as internal signs which give evidence that accelerated aging is occurring. Some of these signs may have triggered your concern already. Take this test to see how rapidly you are aging.

EXCESSIVE AGING TEST

Which of these apply to you (each response worth 1 point)?

1. crow's feet (lines radiating from the eyes)
2. bags under the eyes
3. loss in the elasticity of the skin
4. noticeable thinning of the skin
5. cholesterol deposits on the face and/or eyelids
6. raised brown or flesh-colored spots on the face or hands
7. receding gums

8. age spots (liver spots) on the face, hands, or arms
9. vitilego (white spots due to a loss of pigment on the skin)
10. wrinkle lines on the face radiating from the upper lip toward the nose
11. excessive wrinkling of the face, arms, chest, and/or hands
12. moles that are increasing in number and/or changing in appearance
13. deepening wrinkle lines on the forehead
14. tiny red capillary spots on the face, arms, chest, or legs
15. a noticeable tilting forward of the head and neck
16. nodular growths on the face, nose, hands, or chest
17. loose skin or bags under chin and/or arms
18. stiffening of the spine
19. generalized decrease in joint mobility
20. pain and/or deformity of the joints
21. reduction of the size of the upper lip
22. tendency to shuffle instead of stride while walking
23. ridges on the fingernails
24. increasing occurrence of varicose and/or spider veins
25. gradual (or sudden) decline in visual capacity
26. constant coldness of the hands, feet, arms, legs, face, and/or ears
27. skin that is easily damaged by sunlight
28. dryness of the mucous membranes (nose, vagina, sinuses, mouth, etc.)
29. generalized dryness of the skin
30. one bowel movement or less per day
31. circular lines around the skin of the neck
32. receding hairline or balding (or, in women, massive hair loss)
33. graying of the hair
34. skin tags
35. dryness of the eyes and/or nasal passages
36. persistent tremors
37. heart arrhythmia (irregular heartbeat)
38. rapid heartbeat (80 or more beats per minute)

39. floaters in the eyes
40. loss of muscle tissue in the arms, shoulders, and/or legs
41. Have you noticed a reduction in the size of fingers and/or wrists (i.e. reduced ring size)?
42. Are you becoming increasingly fatigued as the years go on?
43. Are you currently a heavy smoker (one-half pack or more per day)?
44. Have you previously smoked one-half pack or more per day for a period longer than five years?
45. Do you or did you live in the same house as a heavy smoker (who smokes in the house)?
46. Are you currently a heavy drinker (six or more drinks per week)?
47. Had you previously been a heavy drinker for more than five years (six or more drinks per week)?
48. Do you or did you consume large amounts of cane sugar or other refined sugars added to foods or as hidden food additives on a daily or weekly basis?
49. Do you or did you eat deep-fried foods, such as French fries, fried chicken, fried fish, etc., on a daily or weekly basis?
50. Do you or did you regularly consume nitrated and/or preserved meats (hot dogs, ham, bacon, pastrami, bologna, corned beef, salami, jerky, etc.)?
51. Do you currently work or have you in the past worked closely with volatile petrochemicals (e.g. gas station attendants, furniture refinishers, refinery workers, glue workers, road tarring crews, etc.)?
52. Are you exposed to excessive amounts of sunlight without protection (proper clothing, sunscreen)?
53. Are your teeth cracking or chipping?
54. Are you suffering from an increasing degree of muscular weakness?
55. Do you suffer from hearing loss?
56. Do you have a total or near total loss of taste or smell?

57. Do you suffer from macular degeneration, retinopathy, or retinal detachment?
58. Do you suffer from loss of peripheral vision?
59. Are you becoming increasingly vulnerable to injuries (sprains, strains, bruises, cuts, etc.)?
60. Is your hair becoming fine or thin, or is it dull in appearance?
61. Is your recovery time becoming increasingly delayed after becoming ill with colds, flu, or other infections?
62. Do you have a history of heart disease, stroke, and/or hardening of the arteries?
63. Have you been diagnosed with internal cancer?
64. Have you been diagnosed with skin cancer?
65. Have you been diagnosed with osteoporosis?
66. Do you have a history of cataracts?
67. Do you have high blood pressure?
68. Do you have psoriasis and/or eczema?
69. Do you use prescription drugs on a daily basis (if you take 4 or more drugs, add an additional 5 points)?

Your Score _____

---

1 to 11 points *Minimal aging.* The key to preventing further aging is to follow a three-fold approach: improvement in the diet, food restriction, and the intake of the basic antioxidants as an insurance program to retard the aging process. These antioxidants should include 1,000 mg of vitamin C, 400 I.U. of vitamin E, 400 mcg of selenium, 25,000 I.U. of beta carotene, and 1,000 mg of pantothenic acid. Natural-source vitamin C is the ideal form for blocking aging. Instead of the high dose synthetic vitamin C, which according to some studies may, in fact, accelerate aging, take Flavin-C, which is exclusively natural vitamin C plus bioflavonoids, 2 caps twice daily. Additionally, take an iron-free multiple vitamin, as well as additional B-complex. Avoid refined foods such as sugar, white flour, white rice, and commercial vegetable oils. Wild spice extracts are potent antioxidants, far more potent than the typical vitamin pills. By taking them the individual may reduce the amount of antioxidants taken. As a natural and potent antioxidant take Oreganol oil of wild oregano, five drops twice daily. This is a potent and simple way to gain an anti-aging effect.

12 to 28 points *Moderate aging:* Take the antioxidants as described, increasing the daily dosage of beta carotene to 50,000 I.U. and the vitamin E to 800 I.U. In addition, take supplemental antioxidant enzymes, particularly glutathione (300 mg), coenzyme Q-10, riboflavin, and superoxide dismutase (SOD). Natural-source vitamin C is the best form for blocking aging. Instead of the high dose synthetic take Flavin-C, which is exclusively natural vitamin C plus bioflavonoids, 3 caps twice daily. Take an iron-free multiple vitamin plus additional B complex. Reduce your intake of refined sugar, and if you are a smoker, quit before it is too late. Eliminate from the diet all sources of refined vegetable oils. Avoid all nitrated and smoked meats. Curtail or reduce your consumption of alcohol. Wild spice extracts are potent antioxidants, far more potent than the typical vitamin pills. By taking them the individual may reduce the amount of antioxidants taken. As a natural and potent antioxidant take Oreganol oil of wild oregano, five drops twice daily. This is a potent and simple way to gain an anti-aging effect. Apply also an anti-aging skin cream, such as the potent Oreganol cream, to your hands and face on a daily basis.

29 to 42 points *Severe aging:* In addition to the previously mentioned dietary and supplemental advice, take 200 mg of coenzyme Q-10 each day. As aging becomes severe tissue levels of coenzyme Q-10 decline dramatically. Increase the beta carotene dosage to 70,000 I.U., the vitamin C to 3,000 mg, and the vitamin E dosage to 1200 I.U. Take 3,000 mg of pantothenic acid daily. Take this vitamin only in the powdered form, that is the powdered vitamin in capsules. Do not take pressed pills, since they are poorly absorbed. If you are developing large numbers of brown, age, or liver spots, Natural-source vitamin C is the best form for blocking aging. Instead of the high dose synthetic take Flavin-C, which is exclusively natural vitamin C plus bioflavonoids, 3 caps three times daily. Wild spice extracts have recently been shown to be even more powerful than vitamins. In fact, the intake of such extracts reduces the need for megadose vitamin/mineral therapy. Take Oreganol oil of wild oregano, ten or more drops twice daily. ORAC testing, the state of the art in the industry, proves that the active ingredient of Oreganol has among the highest scores known, some 3000 points. This makes it significantly higher in antioxidant power than any food, herb, or vitamin. The oil may also be rubbed topically. Also, consume large amounts of the anti-aging vegetables, a category which includes turnips, radishes, carrots, beets, dark greens, cabbage, broccoli, kale, kohlrabi, onions, artichokes, watercress, and garlic. Apply an anti-aging cream, such as the potent Oreganol antioxidant cream, to the face and hands morning and night. Avoid contact with eyes.

43 and above *Extreme aging:* Warning—aging is occurring at a highly accelerated rate both externally and internally. Follow the aforementioned advice. However, in order to reverse this trend take exceptionally high doses of anti-aging nutrients. In addition, protect your skin from further aging by applying topically the anti-aging nutrients. Supplement your diet with daily doses of the following nutrients:

- vitamin C - 3,000 mg
- vitamin E - 1200 I.U.
- beta carotene - 100,000 I.U.
- thiamine - 100mg
- riboflavin - 100 mg
- pyridoxine - 100 mg
- pantothenic acid - 4000 mg
- organic selenium - 600 mcg

- manganese - 6 mg
- chromium - 600 mcg
- silica - 3000 mg
- calcium - 1200 mg
- magnesium - 800 mg
- potassium - 300 mg
- coenzyme Q-10 - 300 mg
- glutathione (or N-acetyl cysteine) - 500 mg
- fortified royal jelly (i.e. Royal Kick) - 6 caps daily

The last item on this list, fortified royal jelly, is one of the most potent tissue rejuvenating agents known and is significantly more powerful than vitamins C and E. Additionally, daily consume antioxidant enzymes, including glutathione reductase, catalase, peroxidase, and superoxide dismutase. Natural-source vitamin C is the best form for blocking aging. Instead of the high dose synthetic take Flavin-C, which is exclusively natural vitamin C plus bioflavonoids, 3 caps three times daily. Certain herbs and spices, such as garlic, oregano, cumin, coriander, fenugreek, sage, rosemary, and turmeric, possess properties which impede aging. Raw nuts and seeds, particularly almonds, sesame seeds, and sunflower seeds, possess substances which decelerate aging. Load up on foods and spices which block the aging process. Anti-aging fruits include strawberries, cherries, kiwis, papayas, mangoes, and grapefruits. Even more powerful are antioxidant spice extracts. Take Oreganol oil, 20 to 30 drops twice daily. If using the gelcaps, take 4 or more twice daily. Try the Anti-Aging Vegetable Juice Cocktail (see Appendix B). Apply an anti-aging cream, such as the Oreganol antioxidant cream, to exposed skin morning and night, but keep away from eyes.

It is crucial that the diet is altered, since poor dietary habits are the major factors contributing to aging. Processed foods must be replaced by wholesome foods such as fresh fruits, vegetables, nuts, seeds, whole grains, and organic meats. Strictly avoid substances which accelerate aging. These substances include refined sugar, white flour, commercial vegetable and deep-frying oils, alcohol, toxic chemicals (and their fumes), chewing tobacco, and cigarette smoke. If you smoke, stop immediately. If you are exposed to secondhand smoke, make the changes necessary to prevent exposure.

Fasting is also advised, since food abstinence significantly deters the aging process. However, individuals suffering from serious medical conditions must undergo fasts only while under a physician's care.

The Sluggish Thyroid Syndrome

The Sluggish Thyroid Syndrome is perhaps the most commonly occurring hormonal disturbance in America today. It afflicts millions of people of all ages and sexes, although adult women are its usual victims. The thyroid gland controls the metabolic rate and is descriptively known as the "master of metabolism". As many as one in four Americans suffer from reduced thyroid function. Reduced body temperature is perhaps the most common consequence of impaired thyroid function. The individual who wears several extra layers of clothes, wears socks to bed, or who has "ice cold hands" is typically thyroid deficient. The person who abhors the onset of winter is usually thyroid-deficient.

As the master of metabolism the thyroid gland exerts control of several critical functions, including body temperature, digestive enzyme synthesis, stomach acid production, fuel combustion, fat and protein synthesis, white blood cell synthesis and activity, and blood flow. The thyroid gland is also a critical player in the synthesis and activity of sex hormones.

Thyroid disorders are particularly common in the region of North America known as the *goiter belt*. This region was so named because of the high incidence of goiter that occurred there early in this century. Goiter is essentially a pathological enlargement of the thyroid gland. Scientists determined that the states/provinces of the goiter belt had very low iodine levels in their soil and drinking water. Thus, the local food supply was lacking in this critical trace element, and unless an individual regularly consumed seafood, derangement of thyroid function and/or goiter was virtually assured. This "epidemic" was essentially obliterated via the introduction of iodized salt. Even so, goiter, as well as the related condition of thyroid nodules, remains a significant cause of illness in the goiter belt, which includes Ohio, Michigan, Indiana, Illinois, Wisconsin, Ontario, and Manitoba.

THYROID GLAND TEST

Which of these apply to you (each response worth 1 point)?

1. lethargy or weakness
2. tired in the morning and energetic at night
3. dry or coarse hair and/or skin
4. slow or slurred speech
5. swelling of the face and/or eyelids
6. cold hands and feet
7. bloating and indigestion after eating
8. hair loss from the outer third of the eyebrows
9. short-term memory loss
10. depression which is worse in the winter or on overcast days
11. white spots on the fingernails
12. chronic weight problems
13. easily constipated
14. PMS and/or other menstrual difficulties
15. infertility
16. swelling of hands and/or ankles
17. chronic headaches
18. emotionally unstable
19. brittle nails or nails which grow slowly
20. lack of sweating
21. poor appetite and/or lack of hunger
22. hair loss from the scalp, legs, and/or arms

23. generally nervous
24. difficulty getting deep breaths
25. heart palpitations
26. severe muscle cramps, especially at night
27. tendency to bruise easily
28. joint stiffness
29. require prolonged periods to get "warmed up" after exposure to cold
30. excessive appetite (never get full)
31. slow growing hair and/or nails
32. light or heavy menstrual flow
33. brittle hair
34. cholesterol deposits on the face or eyelids
35. lack of sexual desire
36. enlarged facial pores
37. poor hand-to-eye coordination
38. hoarseness or coarse voice
39. inability to translate thoughts into action
40. Do you tend to become depressed in the winter or after exposure to the cold?
41. Do you have a history of ovarian cysts?
42. Do you have repeated breast inflammation and/or infections?
43. Have your periods stopped prematurely?
44. Have you been diagnosed with low stomach acid (hypochlorhydria)?
45. Do you fail to feel rested even after sleeping long hours?
46. Do you have heart disease or hardening of the arteries?
47. Do you have cystic breast disease (lumpy breasts)?
48. Have you noticed that your skin has developed a yellowish tint?
49. Do you have chronic migraine headaches manifested by pain over the bridge of the nose, along the temple, or behind the eyes?
50. Do you drink fluoridated water and/or use fluoridated toothpaste?

51. Do you receive regular fluoride treatments from your dentist, or do you administer them at home?
52. Do you have high cholesterol and/or triglyceride levels?
53. Do you suffer from cracks in the bottom of the heels?
54. Are you morbidly obese, and/or do you have a difficult time losing weight?
55. Do you have a history of repeated miscarriages?
56. Do you have a history of carpal tunnel syndrome?
57. Do you smoke a half pack or more of cigarettes per day?
58. Are you constantly cold, even if you wear extra layers of warm clothing?
59. Do you have a low body temperature (add 2 points for this)?

Your Score _____

---

1 to 11 points *Mildly sluggish thyroid.* Slight imbalances in thyroid function are common and usually can be corrected through dietary means. However, it may be necessary to supplement the diet with thyroid-boosting nutrients such as zinc, copper, magnesium, potassium, tyrosine, B-vitamins, iodine, and vitamin C. Take a multiple vitamin/mineral containing these nutrients. Increase the consumption of foods rich in iodine and reduce the intake of refined/processed foods. Be sure to use sea salt in cooking or sprinkled on foods as a source of iodine. A small dose (1/4 grain or less) of thyroid hormone may be necessary. As a natural iodine and thyroid tonic take ThyroNorm, two caps daily in the morning. This is made with unprocessed wild kelp, which is free of toxic metal residues.

11 to 20 points *Moderately sluggish thyroid.* Severely curtail the consumption of refined sugar, since it causes thyroid burnout. Eat iodine-rich foods and be sure to salt your food with sea salt. Take the following supplements daily: B-complex (1 or 2 tablets), zinc (50 mg), and a multiple vitamin-mineral tablet containing iodine. A prescription of thyroid hormone (1/4 to 1/2 grain) may be necessary. To naturally support thyroid function and as a natural source of iodine and tyrosine take ThyroNorm, four caps daily. This is made with unprocessed wild kelp, which is free of toxic metal residues.

21 to 34 points *Severely sluggish thyroid:* At this level daily thyroid hormone replacement may be necessary. See your doctor and have him/her perform the appropriate blood tests for thyroid function. Be aware that the blood tests can be normal and a thyroid defect may still exist. That is because as much as 70% of thyroid function may be lost before blood tests become abnormal. If the physician suggests thyroid hormone therapy, opt for natural thyroid hormone versus synthetic (e.g. Synthroid), which may be toxic.

Certain substances impair thyroid function. These substances include refined sugar, fluoride, alcohol, hydrogenated fats, and caffeine. Additionally, a number of foods contain substances called goitrogens, which interfere with thyroid function. These anti-thyroid foods include raw cabbage, kale, cauliflower, broccoli, Brussels sprouts, beets, peanuts, almonds, peaches, flax, legumes, beans, carrots, and spinach. What's more, the anti-thyroid components are liberated by juicing. Ironically, the daily consumption of what is regarded to be a healthy food, raw carrot juice, may induce a mild hypothyroid state (Note: cooking inactivates the thyroid-blocking components). In order to reactivate thyroid function, take the following supplements on a daily basis:

- riboflavin - 100 mg daily
- fat-soluble thiamine - 200 mg daily
- niacin - 200 mg daily
- vitamin B-6 - 50 mg daily
- zinc - 50 mg daily
- copper - 3 mg daily
- magnesium - 1,000 mg daily
- natural vitamin C (Flavin-C) - 3 caps twice daily

To naturally support thyroid function and as a natural source of iodine and tyrosine take ThyroNorm, six caps daily. This is made with unprocessed wild kelp, which is free of toxic metal residues.

35 and above *Incompetent thyroid function:* Your thyroid gland is failing to work to any significant degree. To be certain that the symptoms are due to thyroid malfunction take the Broda Barnes underarm thyroid temperature test. This simple at-home test requires only a thermometer. Shake the thermometer down and place it at your bedside. As soon as you awaken put the thermometer under your armpit. Lay motionless in bed for ten minutes and then record the result. Do this for at least ten consecutive days. The newer electronic thermometers require much less time. Women should be aware that their temperatures will naturally rise during menses. The normal underarm temperature is 97.80 or above. If your temperature is consistently below this level, blood tests for evaluating thyroid function are indicated. However, be aware that these tests are often normal even if the thyroid gland is malfunctioning. That is because the tests show only how much thyroid hormone is circulating in the blood and tell nothing of how well the hormones are functioning on a cellular level. Additionally, the loss of up to 70% of thyroid function may occur before blood tests become abnormal. The fact is thousands of Americans have thyroid glands which are operating at 10 to 30% capacity. No wonder so many individuals suffer from chronic fatigue.

If the tests are abnormal, your doctor may suggest thyroid replacement therapy. Insist upon natural thyroid hormone (Armor thyroid, etc.). Do not take Synthroid, it causes bone loss. In addition, the following supplements should be consumed on a daily basis:

- riboflavin - 100 mg
- fat-soluble thiamine - 300 mg
- magnesium - 1,000 mg
- zinc - 50 mg

- copper - 3 mg
- niacin - 250 mg
- vitamin B-6 - 50 mg daily
- natural vitamin C - 4 caps twice daily
- selenium - 400 mcg daily

To naturally support thyroid function and as a natural source of iodine and tyrosine take ThyroNorm, four caps twice daily. This is made with unprocessed wild kelp, which is free of toxic metal residues. It is the most essential thyroid-supporting supplement to take. Also, for those on Synthroid to reverse the bone loss, take Oregamax 3 caps twice daily.

The Adrenal Failure Syndrome

The adrenal glands are the primary organ system for fighting stress. They are responsible for warding off the ill effects of every conceivable mental and/or physical stressor. Emotional strain causes a significant disruption of adrenal function. Anger is perhaps the most devastating of all mental stressors. Researchers have discovered that its negative effects on adrenal function are profound.

Virtually all patients with adrenal insufficiency suffer from severe allergic tendencies. The fact is these glands are the primary means for preventing or reversing allergic reactions. Adrenal failure is frequently associated with hypoglycemia. The adrenal glands exert potent control over blood sugar status. They specifically prevent the levels from dropping suddenly as a result of stress. Individuals with weakened adrenal glands suffer from virtually all of the symptoms of the *Blood Sugar Collapse Syndrome.*

The adrenal glands consist of two sections: an inner portion, known as the *medulla,* and an outer portion, known as the cortex. The medulla produces adrenaline, while the cortex produces a complex array of steroid hormones, descriptively known as *cortical hormones.* The latter category includes cortisone,

DHEA (dihydroepiandosterone), aldosterone, progesterone, estrogen, and testosterone.

The adrenal glands, which are posed atop the kidneys, normally are golf-ball size. As a result of poor nutrition and/or stress, they may become significantly enlarged. This enlargement is due to a phenomenon known as *cellular hypertrophy*. Put simply, the cells within these glands multiply excessively in an attempt to supply the body with the additional steroid hormones demanded by stress. Poor nutrition compromises this process, since a wide range of nutrients are required for adrenal steroid synthesis to proceed normally. The nutrients include fatty acids (especially cholesterol), amino acids, B-vitamins (especially pantothenic acid), vitamin E, vitamin A, vitamin C, bioflavonoids, zinc, selenium, potassium, sodium, manganese, chromium, and magnesium. If the stresses remain unabated and the nutritional deficits are neglected, the adrenal glands ultimately self-destruct and shrink. This is known medically as *atrophy* of the adrenal cortex. When this adrenal atrophy becomes extreme, it may result in a potentially life-threatening condition called *Addison's disease.* In this instance the adrenal glands are totally incapable of producing steroid hormones. Individuals suffering with this condition are unable to cope with stress. Often, the adrenal glands become so weak that even seemingly insignificant stresses can precipitate a decline in health. Then, they are readily attacked, that is because their bodies are in a weakened state. This is why people with weak adrenal glands are highly vulnerable to the development of bizarre infections, including tuberculosis, herpes, hepatitis, and fungal infections.

Tens of millions of Americans suffer from the symptoms of adrenal insufficiency. This condition is rising in incidence every year, largely due to the processed food diet. Severe emotional stress combined with extreme nutritional deficiencies are primary precipitating factors. Stress modification plus improved nutrition usually aids in regenerating the adrenal glands, resulting in return of normal function. When taking this test, having a mirror before you may be helpful.

ADRENAL GLANDS TEST

Which of these apply to you (each response worth 1 point)?

1. constant fatigue
2. muscular weakness
3. sweating or wetness of hands and feet
4. nervousness
5. fainting spells
6. chronic heartburn
7. alternating constipation and diarrhea
8. insomnia
9. low blood pressure
10. blood sugar disturbances
11. mood swings
12. paranoia
13. lightheaded sensation
14. headaches, particularly migraines
15. heart palpitations
16. cravings for salt
17. cravings for sweets
18. intolerance to alcohol
19. intolerance to cigarette smoke and/or exhaust fumes
20. hard pebble-like stools
21. vague indigestion
22. vague abdominal pain
23. vulnerability to food reactions/allergies
24. break out in hives or other rashes
25. clenching and/or grinding of teeth, especially at night
26. lack of appetite
27. infrequent urination and/or lack of thirst
28. premenstrual symptoms (PMS)
29. chronic pain in the lower neck and upper back
30. pain or tightness in the upper neck and/or scalp
31. inability to concentrate and/or confusion
32. panic attacks

33. phobias (agoraphobia, claustrophobia, etc.)
34. easily frustrated
35. compulsive behavior
36. intolerance to hot humid weather (heat exhaustion)
37. intolerance to cold and/or cold hands/feet
38. sense of well being after eating, especially supper
39. depression often relieved by eating
40. difficulty relaxing (unless working)
41. easily distracted
42. tendency to have feelings of guilt
43. extreme sensitivity to odors and/or noises
44. inability to cope with stressful events
45. tendency to cry easily
46. clumsiness
47. hair loss on the outer parts of the lower legs
48. tightness of the armpits
49. Are you unusually ticklish?
50. Do you have upper back pain/tightness, which worsens from stress or cold weather?
51. Do you have a lack of the sensation of fullness after eating?
52. Do you have fine thin hair?
53. Are your lower teeth (lower incisors) crowded, unequal in length, and/or misaligned? (if so, add an additional 2 points)
54. Is your index finger longer than your ring finger? (if so add an additional 4 points)
55. Do you have a tendency to develop yeast or fungal infections?
56. Do you have a breathing disorder, particularly asthma?
57. Do you have an unusually small jaw bone or chin?
58. Have you taken cortisone pills (or prednisone) for prolonged periods (one month or longer)?
59. Do you drink caffeinated beverages on a daily basis?
60. Have you consumed large amounts of refined sugar throughout your life? (if so, add an additional 4 points)

61. Do you consume alcoholic beverages on a daily basis?
62. Do you smoke 1 or more packs of cigarettes daily? (if so, add an additional 3 points)
63. Do you have an excessively low cholesterol level (below 150 mg/dl)?
64. Do you regularly use cortisone creams or ointments?
65. Have you suffered or do you currently suffer from prolonged psychic/emotional stress?
66. Do you suffer from depression and/or weight gain during the winter months?
67. Were you regarded as a "lazy" child?
68. Are you or have you been frequently tormented or ridiculed by others?
69. Do you suffer from or have you suffered from severe infections such as TB, blood poisoning, sepsis or hepatitis?
70. Do you have the initiative and desire to perform tasks but feel physically incapable of doing so?
71. Have you undergone numerous prolonged surgeries?
72. Are you jumpy and/or easily startled?
73. Do you have brown pigment spots about your temples, upper back, or chest?
74. Do you wet the bed or did you previously wet the bed?
75. Do you prefer hot drinks rather than cold drinks, or are you intolerant to cold drinks?

Your Score _____

---

1 to 9 points *Mild adrenal failure:* Even a mild state of adrenal failure can result in significant ill health. To correct this condition avoid substances toxic to the adrenal glands such as refined sugars, caffeine, cocoa, amphetamines, and alcohol. Follow a diet high in protein and natural fat and low in carbohydrates. Take 500 mg of pantothenic acid daily. Additionally, take a multiple vitamin plus minerals and extra vitamin C as natural vitamin C (i.e. Flavin-C) 3 caps twice daily . Salt your food to taste. Also, take a natural adrenal supplement, i. e. AdrenoNorm, four capsules every morning. AdrenoNorm contains royal jelly plus wild sage and wild oregano, which strengthen and balance adrenal function.

10 to 23 points *Moderate adrenal failure:* Warning—the adrenal failure will gradually worsen, that is unless lifestyle and diet are altered. Worry, frustration, anxiety, and depression all create tremendous stress upon the endocrine system, with the adrenal glands bearing the brunt of the damage. Stop mentally battering your adrenal glands or risk falling into total adrenal failure.

The diet should be rich in protein and natural fats and low in sugars and starches. Complex carbohydrates, such as those found in brown rice, wild rice, potatoes, and coarse whole grains, may be well-tolerated by some individuals. However, avoid all dietary sources of refined sugars and curb the consumption of foods naturally rich in sugar such as molasses, honey, fruit juices, oranges, pears, apples, etc.

Take the following supplements in order to preserve your adrenal function and repair any damage that has occurred:

- pantothenic acid - 1,000 mg twice daily
- B-complex - one tablet twice daily
- natural vitamin C - (i.e. Flavin-C) 4 caps twice daily
- tyrosine - 500 mg three times daily
- vitamin A - 15,000 I.U. three times daily
- potassium - 200 mg three times daily
- chromium - 200 mcg three times daily
- Nutri-Sense - 3 heaping tbsp. daily
- Sea salt - as needed in meals (to taste)

Also, take a royal jelly/wild herbal adrenal tonic, i.e. Royal Kick, six caps every morning. This is the most important agent for rebuilding these glands. To eradicate any hidden infections take the germ killing spice oil, that is the Oreganol, 2 gelcaps twice daily or, if using the oil, 10 drops twice daily.

24 to 40 points *Severe adrenal failure:* Beware—complete adrenal collapse is imminent. Lifestyle alterations must occur immediately, i.e. desist from worrying, fretting, grieving, and agitating. Depression and anxiety, as well as fits of anger, devastate adrenal function.

Curtail the consumption of all dietary sources of sugar and strictly adhere to a low-carbohydrate diet. Avoid all sources of alcohol and caffeine. In other words, eat primarily meats, nuts, seeds, olives, cheeses, vegetables, fish, and avocados. Be sure to snack on low-sugar/starch foods between meals to keep the blood sugar stable. Salty snacks such as roasted nuts, pickles, and cheese are ideal. For ideas on snacks and meals see my first book, *How to Eat Right and Live Longer.* In addition, take the following nutritional aids:

- pantothenic acid - 1,000 mg three times daily
- B-complex - 1 tablet three times daily
- natural vitamin C- (i.e. Flavin-C) 4 caps three times daily
- tyrosine - 500 mg twice daily
- vitamin E - 1200 I.U. daily
- vitamin A - 25,000 I.U. twice daily
- magnesium - 400 mg three times daily
- selenium - 200 mcg three times daily
- chromium - 250 mcg three times daily
- manganese - 4 mg three times daily
- potassium - 200 mg daily
- coenzyme Q-10 - 100 mg daily
- carnitine - 1 gram twice daily
- Nutri-Sense - 3 heaping tbsp. daily

Also, take a royal jelly/wild herb-based adrenal tonic, i.e. Royal Kick, four to six caps in the morning and at noon. This is the most important agent for rebuilding these glands. Eat salty snacks and use sea salt in foods. This is perhaps the most critical of all adrenal-supporting supplements.

41 and above *Extreme adrenal failure:* You are in a state of complete adrenal collapse. Perhaps you knew you were ill but didn't realize why. Your adrenal glands are severely damaged, and, as a result, you are unable to cope with the basic elements of life itself. Immediately stop all behaviors and habits which disrupt adrenal function. If you smoke or drink, stop immediately. Curtail the consumption of all stimulants such as caffeine, cocoa, tea, and especially refined sugar. Refined sugar places great stress upon the adrenal glands, increasing the demand for the synthesis of various adrenal hormones. Sugar causes a wastage of adrenal hormones, and this may ultimately lead to internal bleeding within the glands and cellular death.

In order to reverse this pathological condition take the following supplements:

- pantothenic acid - 2,000 mg three times daily
- B-complex - 1 tablet three times daily
- natural vitamin C- (i.e. Flavin-C) 4 caps four times daily
- tyrosine - 500 mg three times daily
- licorice root - 2 capsules twice daily
- vitamin E - 1200 I.U. daily
- vitamin A - 20,000 I.U. twice daily
- magnesium - 400 mg three times daily
- selenium - 200 mcg three times daily
- chromium - 500 mcg three times daily
- vitamin B-6 - 50 mg twice daily
- potassium - 300 mg daily
- bioflavonoids - 2 grams daily
- coenzyme Q-10 - 100 mg twice daily
- carnitine - 1 gram three times daily
- Nutri-Sense - 3 tbsp. daily (as a source of B vitamins)

Also, take a royal jelly/herbal tonic, i.e. AdrenoNorm, five caps twice daily. This is critical for regenerating adrenal function. Royal Kick is a natural source of adrenal steroids, so it is the ideal adrenal support formula. Remember, it took a number of years for the current state of health to develop. Be patient; the adrenal glands will regenerate. However, it may take several months or even years before they heal completely. Be sure to regularly eat salty snacks, and use plenty of sea salt in food. Make sure the sea salt you use has iodine in it to prevent goiter. To eradicate any hidden infections take the germ killing spice oil, that is the Oreganol, 2 gelcaps twice daily or, if using the oil, 10 drops twice daily.

The Blood Sugar Collapse Syndrome

Normally the blood contains sugar in the form of glucose. In fact, glucose is the primary cellular fuel. However, too little or too much sugar in the blood is dangerous. With an excess, diabetes develops. Usually, however, diabetes is preceded by a condition known as *hypoglycemia* or low blood sugar.

Blood sugar disorders are exceedingly common in the United States, with as many as one in two Americans being affected. This is primarily a result of the high sugar diet consumed by the majority of Americans.

The appropriate treatment of this condition is complicated by the fact that physicians are generally unaware that blood sugar disorders are a prevalent cause of ill health. Furthermore, the most accurate method for diagnosing blood sugar disorders, the six-hour glucose tolerance test, is only rarely performed by physicians even if a blood sugar disorder is suspected. To complicate matters the symptoms of blood sugar disorders occur in a wide variety of other illnesses. For example, depression, fatigue, and/or anxiety are among its most common symptoms. For these reasons the Blood Sugar Collapse Syndrome is the most under-diagnosed, as well as mis-diagnosed, of all medical conditions in America today.

The brain consumes a greater amount of sugar for its weight than any other organ. The fact is the brain relies almost exclusively upon sugar, in the form of glucose, as its energy source. As a result, a sudden drop in the blood sugar level may lead to a variety of mental symptoms. Yet, disorientation, anxiety, anger, agitation, depression, and frustration are not the only problems that may arise from hypoglycemia. In fact, rather than developing mental symptoms, some individuals simply fall asleep and/or faint when their blood sugar collapses.

BLOOD SUGAR DISORDER TEST

Which of these apply to you (each response worth 1 point)?

1. mood swings
2. fatigue after eating, worse if dessert is included
3. insomnia (especially waking up after falling asleep)
4. episodes of agitation or temper tantrums
5. dizziness and/or fainting spells
6. legs feel rubbery or weak
7. episodes of shakiness and/or tremors
8. clumsiness
9. headaches (worse after skipping a meal)
10. easily become upset and/or frustrated
11. episodes of cold sweats and/or nausea
12. disorientation
13. depression often relieved by eating
14. sleepiness after eating sugar, fruit, or starch
15. bursts of violent behavior and/or fits of anger
16. attention deficit (or childhood behavioral problems)
17. memory impairment or forgetfulness
18. paranoia and/or anxiety
19. crying spells
20. panic attacks
21. episodes of blurry vision

22. cantankerous behavior
23. sudden drop in energy level during mid-morning or mid-day (if so, add an additional 2 points to your score)
24. nightmares
25. constant worrying
26. indigestion
27. indecisiveness
28. sensations of impending doom
29. poor concentration
30. heart rhythm disturbances
31. uncontrollable negative or self-destructive thoughts
32. episodes of uncontrollable eating (binging)
33. episodes of sudden mental blackouts (if so, add an additional 2 points to your score)
34. Are you accident prone?
35. Do you constantly crave sweets and/or starches?
36. Do you drink alcohol heavily (two or more drinks per day)?
37. Do you consume sweets on a daily basis?
38. Do you have a history of liver and/or pancreatic disease?
39. Do you have a significant family history of diabetes?
40. Do you have chronic migraine headaches?
41. Do you eat fast food on a weekly basis (pizza, hot dogs, hamburgers, subs, doughnuts, etc.)?
42. Do you have intense cravings for salty foods?
43. Do you take birth control pills on a regular basis, or have you done so in the past for two years or more?
44. Have you taken large doses of cortisone, orally or injectable, or do you take it currently on a regular basis?

Your Score _____

1 to 8 points *Mild blood sugar collapse:* If untreated, your blood sugar problems will likely worsen with time. Remove all sources of refined sugars from the diet. Follow a diet rich in protein, natural fats, vegetables, and, to a lesser degree, complex carbohydrates. In addition, take a natural source of B-vitamin, such as Nutri Sense, 2 tablespoons daily. Also take chromium picolinate, 100 mg twice daily.

9 to 22 points *Moderate blood sugar collapse:* Treatment of this mentally and physically debilitating condition requires strict adherence to a low-sugar/starch diet (see *How to Eat Right and Live Longer*). In addition, take the following supplements:

- chromium picolinate - 200 mcg three times daily
- biotin - 1 mg twice daily
- B-complex - 1 tablet twice daily
- zinc - 15 mg three times daily
- magnesium - 400 mg twice daily
- fat-soluble thiamine - 50 mg three times daily
- carnitine - 500 mg twice daily
- Nutri-Sense - 2 heaping tablespoons twice daily
- Oregulin natural blood sugar regulating spice - one
  gelcáp with meals

Note: Oregulin is the key supplement for balancing blood sugar.

Be sure to snack between meals. Safe snacks for blood sugar patients include raw vegetables, nuts, seeds, sliced fresh meats, chicken pieces, plain yogurt, avocados, and cheese. Also, the adrenal glands are involved in blood sugar regulation. To boost adrenal function take Royal Kick, two to four capsules every morning.

23 and above *Severe blood sugar collapse:* Warning—continuous abuse of the body through the consumption of high-sugar foods and other highly processed foodstuffs could result in the onset of diabetes. Curtail the consumption of refined sugar and reduce or eliminate sources of natural sugars such as honey, molasses, orange juice, apple juice, and fruit. Follow the afore-mentioned dietary advice, being sure to snack on high-protein or high-fat foods between meals. In addition, take the following supplements:

- chromium picolinate - 200 mcg three times daily
- manganese chelate - 2 mg three times daily
- B-complex - one tablet twice daily
- multiple mineral - 1 tablet three times daily
- fat-soluble thiamine - 50 mg three times daily
- zinc - 20 mg three times daily
- biotin - 3 mg three times daily
- magnesium - 400 mg twice daily
- carnitine - 1 gram twice daily
- Oregulin blood sugar regulating formula - two gelcaps with each meal

Note: Laboratory tests prove that Oregulin can lower or, in fact, normalize blood sugar. This is a high potency and, therefore, effective formula. Be aware that insulin needs may decline as a result of taking this spice extract. Also, the adrenal glands are involved in blood sugar regulation. Take Royal Kick, four or more capsules every morning.

The Yeast/Fungus Syndrome

Yeast and/or fungal infections have become one of the promi-nent plagues of Western civilization. This is largely a conse-quence of the Western diet. Fungi utilize primarily sugars and starches as their food. Their favorite "dish" is sugar. Fungal growth is greatly enhanced by refined and/or heated sugar, although these organisms also efficiently feed on natural sugars such as those found in fruits and fruit juices.

The rampant use of antibiotics is an additional crucial factor which is responsible for the heightened incidence of yeast infections. Antibiotics kill only bacteria and are particularly aggressive in destroying the body's protective bacteria. This leaves the body vulnerable for colonization by yeasts and fungi.

The mucous membranes of the mouth, sinuses, lungs, intestines, uterus, urethra, and vagina are lined by untold billions of protective bacteria. When these bacteria are destroyed, the tissues are aggressively invaded by various yeast and fungi. This tissue invasion causes severe inflammation. Furthermore, the yeast/fungi produce highly toxic chemicals which disrupt immune function. In fact, the chemicals are so powerful that the immune response against the yeast/fungi is essentially neutralized. Though the mucous membranes are the primary site of damage, chronic fungal infections of the internal organs may occur. The liver, spleen, kidneys, ovaries, thyroid gland, and adrenal glands are all susceptible to infection.

The majority of physicians regard antibiotics as being nontoxic. This is why they prescribe them repeatedly without concern and usually without warning patients of side effects. Patients take numerous doses with seeming impunity. Yet, with each dose, the risk for chronic fungal infections is greatly accelerated. Other drugs which increase the risks for fungal infections include cortisone (especially prednisone), Tagamet, Zantac, antacids, and asthma medications. Tens of millions of Americans consume these drugs every year. Add to this the consumption of antibiotics, and the number of Americans who regularly utilize drugs which enhance fungal growth is in the tens of millions. It should be no surprise that as many as one in four Americans suffer ill health as a consequence of chronic fungal infection.

Fungi also commonly infect the skin. Sites which retain moisture are particularly vulnerable, such as between the toes, the scalp, the groin, and the umbilicus.

YEAST/FUNGUS TEST

Which of these apply to you (each response worth 1 point)?

1. craving for sweets
2. low body temperature
3. indigestion or abdominal discomfort after eating fruits or other sweet foods
4. itching of the vagina, penis, groin, and/or rectum
5. rectal or vaginal burning
6. burning during or after urination
7. vaginal discharge (white, off-white, or cottage-cheesy)
8. skin and/or scalp itches after eating sugar and/or fruit
9. bloating after meals
10. persistent indigestion and/or heartburn
11. itching of the ear canals or umbilicus (belly button)
12. chronic sinus problems
13. intolerance to alcohol
14. sensitivity to chemicals, chemical odors, and/or cigarette smoke
15. seborrhea or heavy dandruff on the scalp, face, or hands
16. ringworm
17. itchy skin and/or scalp
18. reduced white blood count
19. constipation
20. feeling of being in a mental fog
21. chronic diarrhea
22. attention deficit
23. chronic sore or scratchy throat
24. "ice cold" hands or feet
25. severe intolerance to cold weather
26. Do you feel worse on damp humid days?
27. Do you have athlete's foot, toenail, or fingernail fungus?

28. Do you have a history of fungal infection of the internal organs, e.g. lungs, brain, kidneys, bladder, etc.?
29. Do you have a history of eczema and/or psoriasis?
30. Do you have an allergy or sensitivity to airborne molds?
31. Do you have a history of oral, rectal, and/or vaginal thrush?
32. Do you have painful menstrual cramps?
33. Do you have an allergy or sensitivity to moldy and/or fermented foods (blue cheese, aged cheeses, vinegar, soy sauce, brewer's yeast, bakers yeast, etc.)?
34. Do you consume refined sugar on a daily basis?
35. Do you take antibiotics daily, weekly, or monthly?
36. Have you taken ten or more courses of antibiotics (oral or IV) during your lifetime?
37. Do you consume large amounts of "natural sugars" on a daily basis, for instance, orange juice, apple juice, apples, bananas, raisins, pears, dates, prunes, prune juice, canned pineapple, pineapple juice, grape juice, etc.?
38. Do you eat commercially raised meats on a daily basis?
39. Do you have a history of ulcerative colitis or Crohn's disease?
40. Do you have a history of endometriosis?
41. Do you have recurrent urinary tract infections, i.e. bladder infections, urethritis, or pyelonephritis?
42. Do you use steroids (cortisone) on a regular basis (either orally, vaginally, on the skin, or as an inhalant)?
43. Do you use Tagamet, Zantac, and/or antacids regularly?

Your Score ____

---

1 to 8 points *Mild yeast infestation:* Reduce the consumption of refined sugars and restrict the intake of foods naturally high in sugars such as grapes, cherries, orange juice, apple juice, etc. Take an acidophilus supplement and/or eat unsweetened yogurt on a regular basis. Take immune-stimulating nutrients, such as vitamins A, C, E, B-5 and B-6, on a daily basis. As a proven yeast killer take Oreganol oil of wild oregano, five drops under the tongue twice daily or the Oreganol gelcaps, one twice daily.

9 to 17 points *Moderate yeast infestation:* Follow the aforementioned advice. Certain nutrients help stimulate the immune system to destroy the yeast/fungus. The following immune-enhancing supplements are indicated:

* selenium - 500 mcg
* vitamin E - 800 I.U.
* vitamin A - 10,000 I.U.
* biotin - 5 mg
* chromium - 400 mcg
* vitamin C - 1,000 mg
* manganese - 4 mg
* vitamin B-6 - 30 mg
* primrose oil - 6 capsules daily

Additionally, take an acidophilus supplement such as the multiple acidophilus species product, Health-Bac, several times each day (frequent dosages increase the odds for implantation). Raw garlic and onions kill fungal organisms and should be consumed as often as possible. Supplemental garlic is also advised. As a natural yeast killer take Oreganol oil of wild oregano, ten drops twice daily or if taking the gelcaps, two twice daily. Also, in yeast syndromes, thyroid function is usually compromised. Take Thyronorm, 4 caps daily

18 to 25 points *Severe yeast infestation:* Follow the previously mentioned advice regarding diet and supplements. Chronic yeast infections are a significant cause of ill health. Raw garlic and onions should be regularly included in the diet. Eat one clove of raw garlic every day for at least two weeks. Take immune system boosting herbs such as goldenseal and astragalus. In addition, be sure to consume yogurt on a daily basis. As a yeast killer take Oreganol oil of wild oregano, ten drops three times daily or if taking the gelcaps, three twice daily. For tough conditions also take Oregacyn, 2 or more caps twice daily with meals. To strengthen the glands take for the adrenals Royal Kick, 4 caps daily and for the thyroid, Thyronorm, 3 caps twice daily. Thyroid support is crucial in the fungal-destruction process.

26 and above *Extreme yeast infestation:* At this phase of infestation it is possible that internal infection, that is infection of the internal organs, may exist. Destroy the yeasts with immunotherapy by taking the following nutrients:

- vitamin A - 10,000 I.U.
- selenium - 800 mcg
- zinc - 70 mg
- vitamin C - 4,000 mg
- vitamin E - 800 I.U.
- chromium - 400 mcg
- magnesium - 4 mg
- biotin - 5 mg
- riboflavin - 50 mg
- vitamin B-6 - 50 mg
- folic acid - 10 mg

In addition, there are a host of herbs and other natural substances which kill fungi. They include oil of wild oregano, aloe, goldenseal root, tannic acids, mathake, and Pau D'arco, any or all of which may pose helpful additions to the anti-yeast protocol. As a natural yeast killer take Oreganol oil of wild oregano, 20 drops three times daily or if taking the gelcaps, 3 to 4 caps three times daily. For tough cases also take the Oregacyn, 2 to 3 caps twice daily with meals. To strengthen the glands take for the adrenals Royal Kick, 6 caps daily and for the thyroid, ThyroNorm, 4 caps twice daily. Thyroid support is crucial in the fungal-destruction process.

Intestinal Parasite Syndrome

This is an exceedingly common syndrome, afflicting untold millions of Americans and hundreds of millions of people worldwide. Parasites may be defined as microbes which infect or "live off of" human tissue. The primary categories are *protozoans* and *helminths*. The protozoans include amoebas, giardia, and trichomonas. The helminths include the various worms such as roundworms, pinworms, hookworms, and tapeworms.

The major distinction between parasites and bacterial viruses is that the former are larger and in some instances may become so large that they are visible with the naked eye. In contrast, bacteria and viruses can be seen only with the aid of a microscope. What makes parasites particularly dangerous is that they can infect people via three forms: the live organism itself, its eggs, or its cysts.

Parasitic illnesses are a major plague of modern society. Both acute and chronic diseases may result from parasitic infections. Acute diseases include flu syndromes, hepatitis, food poisoning, diarrheal illness, appendicitis, and gallbladder attacks. Chronic diseases include anemia, colitis, intestinal ulcers, liver disease (including cirrhosis), arthritis, immune defects, and lung disease.

The "Milwaukee Parasite" crisis of 1993 is just one example of the enormity of this problem. In April 1993, this city's water supply was contaminated with a parasite called *cryptosporidium*. Apparently, the organism and/or its cysts are resistant to chlorine. It is estimated that some 400,000 people, or one-half of the city's population, were infected; several died.

Parasites are often difficult to kill. The key is to stimulate the immune response against them. Additionally, various herbs are anti-parasitic, including black walnut extract, ginger root, echinacea, grapefruit seed extract, raw pumpkin seeds, garlic, oil of oregano, oil of fennel, oil of cumin, and onion extract.

INTESTINAL PARASITE TEST
(each response worth 1 point)

Do you experience:

1. rectal itching
2. rectal pressure
3. muscular wasting and/or weakness
4. chronic vague abdominal pain
5. ravenous appetite
6. bloating, especially after eating
7. weight loss or inability to gain weight
8. constant or frequent heartburn
9. diarrhea
10. mucous in stools
11. night sweats
12. insomnia
13. severe fatigue
14. nausea and/or vomiting
15. fever and/or chills
16. constant belching
17. stomach pain after eating
18. poorly formed stools
19. itchy skin, worse at night
20. dark circles under the eyes
21. colon pain
22. ulcerative colitis or Crohn's disease (add an additional 2 points for each)
23. Have you traveled frequently overseas and/or to Mexico?
24. Have you ever developed diarrheal disease or severe fever while traveling abroad?
25. Do you frequently eat raw or smoked fish (sushi)?
26. Do you eat prosciutto and/or home-made sausages?
27. Do you own house dogs that you often handle, pet, or kiss?
28. Did you live overseas before becoming a U.S. resident?

29. Have you ever lived in a tropical region?
30. Do you drink untreated and/or unfiltered water in the wilderness or when traveling overseas?
31. Do you fail to wash your hands carefully after using the restroom?
32. Do you tend to experience digestive distress after eating fatty foods?
33. Do you have a long-term history of chronic anemia (low blood count)?
34. Do you suffer from persistent joint pain?
35. Are you a restless sleeper?

Your Score _____

---

1 to 5 points *Mild parasitic infestation:* Certain symptoms of parasitic infection are nonspecific. Thus, at this level the symptoms could be due to a variety of other illnesses or infections. As a trial to determine if you have parasites eat 2 or 3 cloves of raw garlic daily. Or, take a multiple spice extract, such as Oregacyn, 2 capsules twice daily. If the symptoms improve within one week, parasitic infestation is virtually confirmed. Oreganol oil of wild oregano is also an excellent antiparasitic.

6 to 13 points *Moderate parasitic infestation:* Medical tests for determining the presence of parasites are indicated. Eat two cloves of raw garlic three times daily, ideally on an empty stomach *(Note:* Some individuals cannot tolerate this and should consume it only with meals.) If the symptoms improve, continue consuming 2 cloves three times daily for two weeks. Ideally, take the garlic while on a gallbladder liver flush. The liver is a primary site of infestation, and the flush helps drive parasites from the liver into the bowels so that the garlic can destroy them. The flushing agent is a mixture of 1/4 to 1/2 cup of extra virgin olive oil (or pure rice bran oil) combined with several tablespoonfuls of vinegar or lemon juice. To this add the potent spice extract mixture, Liva Clenz, 5 droppersful; drink a quarter cup of this mixture daily. This will greatly aid both in flushing out the parasite and in liver cell regeneration. The flush should be performed for five to seven days. During this period follow an exclusively high fat diet; your menu will consist of fatty foods such as eggs, cheese, butter, beef, lamb, avocados, olives, nuts, and seeds. Salads are allowed as are the following liver-cleansing fruits and vegetables:

- black radish root
- daikon and red radish
- apple or pear skins (pectin binds toxins generated from the flush)
- turnips
- onions, garlic, leeks, shallots, parsley, and watercress
- capers
- Jerusalem artichoke

Capers aid in liver regeneration; be sure to top your salads with them. Onions, garlic, turnips, and radishes are anti-parasitic in addition to being stimulants of biliary flow. However, the secret to the success of this flush is the olive oil and high-fat diet, since fat purges the liver of the bile and the parasites that live within it. To aid in the flush take Gene's wild greens, five droppersful daily. Additionally, raw pumpkin seeds are anti-parasitic. Consume at least three large handfuls daily during the liver flush. Ginger root also possesses significant anti-parasitic activity: take 3 capsules three times daily on an empty stomach. Fresh ginger may also be used. As a potent, natural antiparasitic agent take Oregacyn, 2 caps twice daily. Oreganol oil of wild oregano is also an excellent antiparasitic.

14 to 21 *Severe parasitic infestation:* Follow the advice listed previously. To aid in the flush take Gene's wild greens, five to ten droppersful daily. In addition, increase the garlic consumption during the liver flush to 4 cloves three times daily. Eat raw onions as often as possible. Take the various anti-parasitic herbs recommended previously and consume at least four handfuls of raw pumpkin seeds each day. Raw pumpkin seeds contain a substance which kills intestinal worms. A thymus glandular supplement (6 to 9 capsules), zinc (75 mg), and selenium (400 mcg) are crucial nutrients which provoke the anti-parasitic immune response. As a potent antiparasitic agent take Oregacyn, 3 caps twice daily. This is among the most effective natural antiparasitic agents known. Oreganol oil of wild oregano is also a potent antiparasitic: take 10 drops twice daily.

23 and above *Extreme parasitic infestation:* Warning: this is a significant dilemma. The fact is chronic extreme parasitic infection greatly increases the risk for a variety of diseases, including cancer, heart disease, stroke, diabetes, and arthritis. Follow the aforementioned advice. To aid in flushing out the parasites and toxins take Gene's Wild Greens, five droppersful twice daily. In addition, during the liver flush increase the garlic consumption to 3 cloves three times daily. Eat raw onions as often as possible. Take the various anti-parasitic herbs recommended previously and consume at least four handfuls of raw pumpkin seeds each day. Raw pumpkin seeds contain a substance which kills intestinal worms. A thymus glandular supplement (6 to 9 capsules), zinc (75 mg), and selenium (400 mcg) are crucial nutrients which provoke the anti-parasitic immune response. As a potent antiparasitic agent take Oregacyn, 3 caps twice daily. This is among the most effective natural antiparasitic agents known, far more potent than black walnut or cloves, Oreganol (oil of wild oregano) is also a potent antiparasitic: using the maximum strength variety take 20 drops twice daily.

Chronic Viral Infestation

This test is highly accurate for indicating the existence of chronic viral infestation. In other words, virtually any chronic viral infection can be determined through it. This is because regardless of the organism chronic viral infections are similar in their presentation.

Viral infections are a major cause of disease. The problem is most people are unaware they are suffering from them. Viruses can disrupt the health of virtually any organ, causing particularly diseases of the liver, immune system, spleen, brain, spinal cord, intestines, and bone marrow.

CHRONIC VIRAL INFESTATION TEST
Which of these apply to you (each response worth 1 point)?

1. constant fatigue unrelieved by sleeping
2. muscles are extremely weak
3. highly vulnerable to colds/flu
4. can't mount a strong defense against infection
5. break out in cold sores often
6. frequent sore throats
7. body temperature fluctuations
8. numbness and tingling of the legs, feet, arms, or hands
9. muscular paralysis
10. canker sores
11. memory loss
12. dementia (senility)
13. work in a medical laboratory
14. work in a high rise building
15. work in a day care center
16. persistent spasms or "locking" of back, neck, and/or spinal muscles
17. muscles are spastic
18. persistent spinal pain
19. feel sleepy constantly
20. no desire for sexual activity
21. feel fatigued or sick from exercise
22. warts

23. poor wound healing
24. skin tags
25. consume refined sugar on a daily or weekly basis
26. stress load is high
27. one or more blood transfusions
28. Do you allow the dog to lick your face, or do you kiss it?
29. Do you suffer from hepatitis?
30. Have you been diagnosed with Epstein-Barr syndrome or CMV?
31. Do you suffer from multiple sclerosis?
32. Do you suffer from AIDS or HIV (add an additional 5 points)?
33. Do you have a low white blood cell count (below 5.0)?
34. Are you a health care worker who works in a hospital?
35. Are you a health care worker who works in a clinic?
36. Do you work around or with radioactive chemicals?
37. Have you been diagnosed with a weak or enlarged heart muscle (cardiomyopathy)?
38. Are you a strict vegan?
39. Do you eat large amounts of commercial poultry?
40. Do you eat commercial eggs on a daily basis?
41. Do you suffer from shingles?
42. Is the protein level in your blood low (i.e. a low albumin or globulin)?
43. Do you suffer from leukemia?
44. Do you feel flu-ish (even though you don't have the flu)?
45. Do you have night sweats?
46. Have you developed a chronic illness after a severe bout with the flu?
47. Do you suffer from Bell's palsy?
48. Do you suffer from chronic fatigue syndrome?
49. Are you taking immuno-suppressive drugs, like

cortisone, Prednisone, methotrexate, etc. on a daily
or regular basis?
50. Are you currently undergoing chemotherapy?

Your Score _____

1 to 7 points *Possible/probable viral infestation syndrome:* Viral
infestation is chronic and, thus, its existence may be difficult to
determine. If you scored 6 or 7, you have a possible hidden
chronic virus infection. To correct the condition take anti-viral
spice extracts, like oil of oregano, oil of cinnamon, and oil of
clove. Or, take an immune boosting spice mix, like Vira Clenz, 5
drops twice daily under the tongue or in juice/water. Take also
crude wild oregano capsules, like Oregamax, two capsules twice
daily. Eat hefty amounts of garlic and onion in food. Avoid
refined sugar and alcohol, as both of these substances weaken
immunity, increasing the risks for viral invasion. In order to keep
further viruses from invading your body be sure to take the oil of
wild oregano and Oregamax daily.

8 to 14 points *Significant viral infestation syndrome:* A score
of 8 or more indicates a high likelihood of a hidden chronic
viral infection. To correct the condition take anti-viral spice
extracts, like oil of oregano, oil of cinnamon, and oil of clove.
Preferably, take a Vira Clenz drops, which contains a combination of such spice oils, 20 drops twice daily under the
tongue or in juice/water (note: this may be only available via
mail order: 1-800-243-5242 or, internationally, 1-847-473-
4700/droregano@hotmail.com). Take Oreganol (oil of wild
oregano), 5 drops under the tongue twice daily. Siddiqui, pub-
lishing in Medical Science Research, determined that oil of
oregano disintegrated difficult-to-kill viruses, like herpetic
viruses. Take also wild oregano oil capsules, two caps twice
daily. Eat hefty amounts of garlic and onions in food. Avoid

refined sugar and alcohol, as both of these substances weaken immunity, increasing the risks for viral invasion. Research by major universities proves that the oil of wild oregano kills germs quickly and is even more effective than certain antibiotics. Certainly, for viruses, which are immune to antibiotics, oil of oregano is a potent killer. Plus, it is non-toxic, whereas anti-viral drugs present significant toxicity. Never take generic forms of oil of oregano,which are usually from the potentially toxic Thymus Capitus.

15 to 22 points *Extensive viral infestation syndrome:* This score indicates a high likelihood of a hidden chronic virus infection. To boost immunity take the anti-viral spice extract, Vira Clenz, 40 drops twice daily under the tongue or in juice/water (see previous section for availability). Take Oreganol, 10 drops under the tongue twice daily or take it as gelcaps, 3 caps twice daily. Note: to be safe the oregano oil must always be the type emulsified in extra virgin olive oil. Take also crude wild oregano capsules, like Oregamax, three capsules twice daily. Eat hefty amounts of garlic and onions in food. Also, consume anti-viral nutrients, that is nutrients which greatly boost immune function. These nutrients include selenium, pantothenic acid, vitamin B-6, vitamin C, and vitamin A. A crude natural source vitamin C may be desired. Natural source vitamin C is functionally and structurally unique compared to the synthetic. Take a 100% natural source vitamin C, like Flavin-C, 3 to 4 capsules twice daily. To boost blood flow and strengthen the arteries take crude red grape powder i.e. Resvitanol powder, one teaspoon twice daily. Avoid refined sugar and alcohol, as both of these substances weaken immunity, increasing the risks for viral invasion. In order to prevent further viral invasion be sure to take the oil of wild oregano and Vira Clenz on a daily basis. Note: Never take generic forms of oil of oregano, which are usually from the potentially toxic, Thymus capitus. Such oils are often heavily refined and/or they are derived from non-edible species. Use only oregano spice oil, which is safe for all ages. When purchasing, look for the distinction P73, which is the researched, tested and spice oil type of wild oregano oil. P73 is fully safe for human and animal use.

22 to 30 points *Extreme viral infestation syndrome:* This indicates an extremely high likelihood of a hidden chronic virus infection. To correct the condition follow the aforementioned advice. Take the anti-viral spice extract like Vira Clenz, 40 drops three or more times daily under the tongue or in juice/water. Take oil of wild oregano, 20 drops under the tongue three times daily. Note: to be safe the oregano oil must always be the type emulsified in extra virgin olive oil. Take also crude wild oregano capsules, four capsules twice daily. Eat hefty amounts of garlic and onion in food. Also, consume anti-viral nutrients, that is nutrients which greatly boost immune function. These nutrients include selenium, pantothenic acid, vitamin B-6, vitamin C, and vitamin A. A crude natural source vitamin C may be desired. Natural source vitamin C is functionally and structurally unique compared to the synthetic. Take a 100% natural source vitamin C, like Flavin-C, 3 to 4 capsules twice daily. Avoid refined sugar and alcohol, as both of these substances weaken immunity, increasing the risks for viral invasion. Never take generic oil forms of oil of oregano,which are usually from the potentially toxic, *Thymus capitus.*

31 and above *Monumentally extreme viral infestation syndrome:* Viral infestation is difficult to determine with blood tests. However, this score indicates the existence of a massive internal viral infestation. Since it is chronic, it may be impossible to determine the exact type of virus. However, the key is to greatly assist the immune system in cleansing the virus from the system. To correct the condition take anti-viral spice extracts, like oil of oregano, oil of cinnamon, and oil of clove. Or, take an immune boosting spice mix, like Vira Clenz drops, 40 or more drops four or more times daily under the tongue or in juice/water. Take oil of wild oregano, 10 to 20 drops under the tongue three times daily. Preferably, take the SuperStrength variety, 15 to 20 drops twice daily. Note: to be safe the oregano oil must always be the type emulsified in extra virgin olive oil. Take also crude wild oregano capsules, like Oregamax, four to six capsules twice daily. Selenium and zinc offer immune support by aiding the white cells' ability to destroy viruses; take respectively 600 mcg and 75 mg daily of each. Also, take natural source vitamin A, 10,000 I.U. daily. Pantothenic acid and vitamin B-6 are immune boosting: take 1000 mg of absorbable pantothenic acid and 100 mg of coenzyme B-6 (P5P) daily. Take a crude natural vitamin C/bioflavonoid formula. The vitamin C boosts antiviral defenses by increasing the synthesis of immunoglobulins and interferon and the bioflavonoids strengthen cells, blocking viral invasion—take Flavin-C, 4 capsules twice daily. Oil of wild Rosemary in extra virgin olive oil offers anti-viral support: take 20 drops under the tongue twice daily. Also, take the Vira Clenz internally, 10 drops twice daily with meals. Eat hefty amounts of garlic and onion in food. Avoid refined sugar and alcohol, as both of these substances weaken immunity, increasing the risks for viral invasion. Also, avoid the intake of hydrogenated oils, like margarine; these oils impair the ability of white blood cells to destroy viruses. Note: Oreganol (oil of oregano) and crushed wild oregano capsules have no known side effects that could damage the tissues, whereas anti-viral drugs are potentially caustic, with numerous side effects. Be aware that this is not medical advice, but is for informational purposes. See your doctor for any medical complaint. Never take generic forms of oil of oregano, which are usually from the potentially toxic, *Thymus capitus*.

The Inappropriate Estrogen Syndrome

Estrogen is regarded as essential to womanhood itself. While it is possible for women to live without it, the quality of their lives is usually compromised. However, estrogen deficiency is only one aspect of this dilemma. That is because many women have enough estrogen but suffer from a metabolic defect where they fail to utilize it properly. Other women produce an excess of estrogen, that excess being toxic. Abnormally high estrogen levels are associated with breast, uterine, and ovarian cancer in addition to less serious conditions such as cystic ovaries and fibrocystic breast disease. Oddly, the symptoms of too little, too much, and poorly utilized estrogen are similar, as is represented by this test.

ESTROGEN TEST
Which of these apply to you (each response worth 1 point)?

1. night sweats
2. hot flashes
3. breast engorgement, worse during or before periods
4. insomnia
5. mood swings, worse during or before periods
6. heavy menstrual bleeding
7. excessive or painful menstrual cramps
8. dryness of the vaginal membranes
9. poor vaginal lubrication
10. PMS
11. loss of libido
12. Do you have a family history of breast cancer?
13. Do you currently have breast cancer, or did you have it in the past (add an additional 2 points)?
14. Do you have a history of endometriosis?
15. Do you have a family history or current history of uterine fibroids?
16. Do you have a family history or current history of ovarian cysts?
17. Do you have a family history or current history of ovarian cancer?
18. Do you have a family history or current history of fibrocystic breast disease?

19. Do you take birth control pills?
20. Have you taken birth control pills for 5 or more years in the past?
21. Have you undergone a complete or partial hysterectomy?
22. Do you become weak or tired prior to or during menses?
23. Do you suffer from headaches occurring prior to or during menses?
24. Do you suffer from hirsutism (i.e. excessive hair growth), especially on the face?
25. Do you maintain excessive amounts of weight in your hips and/or breasts?
26. Do you suffer from chronic liver disease?
27. Do you consume refined sugar on a daily or weekly basis?
28. Do you consume margarine, refined vegetable oils, and/or deep-fried foods on a daily basis?
29. Do you consume alcohol and/or caffeine on a daily basis?
30. Do you have a history of infertility and/or repeated miscarriages?
31. Do you adhere to a strict low-fat diet?
32. Have you had an abnormal pap smear, or do you suffer from cervical dysplasia?

Your Score _____

---

1 to 6 points *Mild estrogen imbalance:* This low-level imbalance is probably due to a metabolic defect rather than a deficiency/excess. The metabolism of estrogen is controlled by the liver, ovaries, and adrenal glands, and it is likely that the function of these organs is impaired. Additionally, B-vitamins help regulate estrogen synthesis and metabolism. To correct this imbalance take a B-complex supplement, along with a natural source of B-vitamins such as Nutri-Sense. Contrary to popular belief the diet should be rich in natural fats as well as cholesterol. Estrogen is a cholesterol molecule and, thus, dietary cholesterol is an important resource for its synthesis. In addition, take 5 mg of folic acid each day, since this B-vitamin is the primary one for regulating estrogen synthesis. As a source of natural, safe estrogens and estrogen balancing herbs take EstroNorm, 4 capsules every morning. Avoid refined sugar, alcohol, and caffeine. What's more, strictly avoid the consumption of refined oils. The latter fully disrupt hormone metabolism. Plus, the refined vegetable oils are potent carcinogens.

7 to 13 points *Moderate estrogen imbalance:* Follow the previously mentioned advice. In addition, take large doses of the nutrients which stimulate and/or regulate estrogen production, as follows:

- folic acid - 5 to 10 mg
- riboflavin - 50 mg
- vitamin B-6 - 50 mg
- choline - 1 gram
- magnesium - 800 mg
- pantothenic acid - 1 gram
- vitamin E - 1200 I.U.
- vitamin A - 25,000 I.U.

Also, as a natural source of non-toxic estrogen and progesterone, as well as estrogen balancing herbs, take EstroBalance, 4 caps every morning. What's more, strictly avoid the consumption of refined oils. The latter fully disrupt hormone metabolism. Plus, the refined vegetable oils are potent carcinogens.

14 and above *Severe estrogen imbalance:* At this level of imbalance estrogen replacement therapy may be indicated. However, most estrogenic drugs are toxic, and evidence exists that women who take them over prolonged periods have a higher risk for breast and/or uterine cancer. Estriol is a nontoxic form of estrogen but is not readily available from traditional pharmacies. The solution may be to take herbs which stimulate the production of estrogen as well as the vitamins that increase its synthesis. Follow the aforementioned advice, increasing the dose of panthothenic acid to one gram twice daily and folic acid to 10 mg daily. Strictly avoid the intake of caffeine, refined sugar, alcohol, and refined vegetable oils. Herbs which aid in the balancing of estrogen levels include rosemary, sage, oregano, and black cohosh. A formula containing all such herbs has become recently available. For more information call 1-800-243-5242.

Note: The symptoms of Inappropriate Estrogen Syndrome may be due primarily to progesterone deficiency. A deficiency of this hormone occurs most commonly premenstrually. As a natural source of non-toxic progesterone and estrogen balancing herbs, take EstroBalance, 4 to 6 capsules every morning. Royal jelly is a top source of naturally occurring estrogens and progesterone. What's more, EstroBalance provides the full spectrum of adrenal and female steroids, some 55 in total. This means that royal jelly is the ideal natural steroid/hormone supplement. Regardless of whether high or low it helps balance the hormone status.

The Liver Dysfunction Syndrome

The liver is the body's workhorse, performing a greater number of functions than any other organ. In particular, it is responsible for the detoxification of any external poisons as well as those produced within the body. Diseases of the liver are rising greatly in incidence. Such diseases include liver cancer, hepatitis, Gilbert's disease, liver abscesses, parasitic infestation, diabetes, and cirrhosis.

Alcoholism is rampant, and as many as 30 million Americans suffer liver damage as a result of constant abuse. Alcoholics constitute a greater number of addicted individuals than heroin, marijuana, cocaine, and prescription drug addicts combined.

Alcoholics suffer immensely as a result of chronic consumption. A single alcoholic drink kills as many as a million liver cells as well as brain cells. This explains why alcohol is the number one cause of liver disease. Yet, extensive damage is inflicted upon other organs as well. Alcohol is a primary cause of hypertension, stroke, pancreatic disease, and heart disease as well as numerous types of cancer.

Long-term consumption of alcohol causes extensive liver damage, ultimately resulting in hepatitis and cirrhosis. Hepatitis is a potentially life-threatening disease. Alcohol consumption is one of many causes of hepatitis. Infectious hepatitis may develop as a result of inappropriate hygiene and sanitation, the consumption of foul water, or food contamination (for instance, shellfish contaminated by water-borne feces). Chemical hepatitis may occur as the result of drug/alcohol addiction, toxic chemical exposure poisoning, and drug reactions. Additionally, hepatitis can be transmitted during sex and, in fact, occurs most commonly in the sexually promiscuous. The fact is regarding hepatitis C sexual promiscuity is one of the major causes. Blood transfusions are another major cause.

The liver marshals several essential functions. It acts as the primary storage depot for nutrients: vitamins, minerals, antioxidants, and co-enzymes. The synthesis of various proteins occurs primarily in the liver, including crucial antioxidant enzymes such as glutathione and superoxide dismutase. It is the primary organ which makes the various cellular enzymes. Additionally, it aids in the metabolism of a variety of hormones, including thyroid hormone, estrogen, and adrenal steroids. Finally, the liver is the primary organ responsible for the detoxification and decomposition of molecular compounds, whether natural or synthetic. For instance, it is the only organ which can efficiently rid the body of the breakdown products of commonly consumed substances, such as alcohol, drugs, fat-soluble vitamins, preservatives, artificial colors/flavors and/or hormones.

All obese individuals suffer from impaired liver function. That is because the liver is the first internal organ to become infiltrated with fat. The fat is deposited within the liver cells, which are known as *hepatocytes,* greatly impairing their ability to function. In the extreme this fat infiltration causes degeneration of the liver cells. Usually, when the weight is lost the liver cells regenerate and function returns to normal. In addition, certain nutrients, notably biotin, lipoic acid, thiamine, inositol, choline, and methionine, aid in liver cell regeneration by reversing fatty liver. Herbal tonics which help purge the liver of fat include the crude wild greens (i.e. the Gene's powerdrops) and spice oil complexes such as LivaClenz.

This exam is applicable to those suffering from extensive liver disease as well as individuals whose livers simply are not working up to speed. The liver is the human body's primary detoxification organ, and it processes billions of molecules of noxious agents every hour of every day. Therefore, it is crucial to keep the liver in an optimal state of health.

LIVER DYSFUNCTION TEST
Which of these apply to you (each response worth 1 point)?

1. intolerance to alcohol
2. intolerance to sugar
3. tendency to gain weight easily
4. blood sugar disturbances
5. pale, greasy stools that float
6. chronic indigestion unrelieved by antacids
7. intolerance to fatty foods and/or cooking oils
8. foul-smelling bowel gas
9. sensitivity to chemical fumes (exhaust fumes, diesel fumes, perfumes, etc.)
10. high cholesterol and/or triglycerides (or excessively low cholesterol - below 140 mg/dl)
11. persistent sleepiness (narcolepsy) and/or fatigue
12. sudden hair loss
13. right-sided upper abdominal pain
14. chronic itching (pruritus)
15. dark circles and/or bags under the eyes

16. Do you consume alcohol regularly (4 or more drinks per week)?
17. Are you 20 or more pounds overweight?
18. Do you have a history of hepatitis and/or cirrhosis?
19. Do you have a history of intestinal or hepatic parasites?
20. Do you consume Tylenol on a daily or weekly basis?
21. Has your gallbladder been removed, and/or do you have a history of gallstones?
22. Do you have chronic constipation (fewer than one bowel movement per day)?
23. Do you take two or more prescription medications on a daily basis?
24. Have you in the past or do you currently use recreational or hard drugs (marijuana, cocaine, heroine, etc.)?
25. Have you received or are you currently receiving chemotherapy treatments?
26. Are you taking cholesterol-lowering medications?
27. Do you work with or near toxic chemicals, or have you worked with them in the past?
28. Do you have elevated bilirubin and/or liver enzymes?
29. Do you have a history of impaired immunity and/or immune deficiency?
30. Do you have thick ridges on the fingernails?
31. Do you take birth control pills, or have you taken them for one year or longer in the past?
32. Do you have a low blood globulin level?
33. Are you a diabetic, or do you have a significant family history of diabetes?
34. Do you have a tendency to bleed excessively (poor blood clotting)?
35. Do you have giardia infection, intestinal worms, or amoebic dysentery?

Your Score ____

1 to 7 points *Mild liver dysfunction:* Mild dysfunction of the liver can usually be resolved through dietary means and by the avoidance of toxic compounds. Certainly, in order to have a disease-free liver alcohol must be strictly avoided as well as refined sugar. Increase the consumption of liver-detoxifying foods such as onions, garlic, leeks, shallots, capers, radishes, turnips, dark greens, squash, and pumpkin. Avoid all synthetic drugs. As a general liver cleanser take Oregacyn Liver formula, 1 capsule with a fatty meal daily. Or, take it with two tablespoons of extra virgin olive oil.

8 to 14 points *Moderate liver dysfunction:* The liver is the human body's manufacturing plant. It is crucial to optimize liver function to prevent disease and improve health. Avoid direct contact with toxic compounds in or around the home or at work. Sugar tends to impair liver function. Thus, high carbohydrate foods, such as pasta, breads, sweets, and bakery, should be avoided. Hydrogenated oils impair liver function. Avoid them entirely. Consume foods which aid in liver detoxification such as ginger root, parsley, parsley root, radishes, watercress, cilantro, and onions. In addition to dietary changes, take the following supplements:

- beet juice tablets or powder
- Gene's Wild Greens - 40 drops daily
- organic selenium - 300 mcg daily
- beta carotene - 25,000 I. U. daily
- fat-soluble thiamine - 200 mg daily
- choline and methionine - 1 gram of each daily
- acidophilus and bifidus - 2 capsules of each twice daily
- biotin - 3 mg twice daily

Plus, take Oregacyn Liver, 4 capsules daily with a quarter cup of extra virgin olive oil. Strictly avoid the intake of alcohol, refined sugar, and drugs.

15 to 21 points *Severe liver dysfunction:* Follow the afore-mentioned advice. It is crucial to change dietary habits imme-diately. Refined vegetable oils, margarine, partially hydro-genated fats, and refined sugars are all hepatotoxic. Curtail the consumption of alcoholic beverages, and, if you are tak-ing drugs, do everything possible to reduce the dosage. Preferably, work with your doctor to eliminate them. Additionally, follow the gallbladder and liver flush suggested in the section on parasitic infestation. Take the following sup-plements on a daily basis:

- beet juice powder or tablets
- selenium - 500 mcg
- beta carotene - 50,000 I.U.
- vitamin E - 800 I.U.
- choline and methionine - 500mg of each
- biotin - 5 mg twice daily
- inositol - 1 gram twice daily
- vitamin C - 2,000 mg
- ginger - 6 capsules
- acidophilus and bifidus - 3 capsules with meals
- Oregacyn Liver multiple spice formula–3 caps twice daily
- Gene's Green Powerdrops (a potent liver tonic) -
  40 drops twice daily (Note: take the Powerdrops
  and Oregacyn Liver with extra virgin olive oil to stimulate
  the gallbladder 'flush' reflex).

22 and above *Extreme liver dysfunction:* Warning—continued exposure to toxic chemicals, drugs, or alcoholic beverages may cause irreparable liver damage. Blood tests for determining liver function are definitely indicated.

Follow the previously mentioned dietary advice. Drink no alcohol. Consume foods which stimulate the healing processes within the liver. Examples include black and daikon radishes, onions, garlic, leeks, turnips, beets, watercress, parsley, raw nuts, seeds, ginger, turmeric, and capers. Try the Gingerized Liver Regeneration Drink in the recipe section (see Appendix B). In addition, take the following liver-repairing supplements on a daily basis:

- beet juice tablets or powder
- selenium - 600 mcg
- choline and methionine - 1 gram of each
- biotin - 10 mg twice daily
- inositol - 2 grams twice daily
- vitamin E - 1200 I.U.
- silymarin - 1 gram
- black radish root - 8 capsules
- beta carotene - 50,000 I.U.
- ginger - 9 capsules daily
- fat-soluble thiamine - 500 mg
- vitamin C - 2,000 mg
- Oregacyn Liver formula (multiple spice) - 3 caps twice daily
- stabilized acidophilus and bifidus (i.e. Health-Bac) 1 to 2 teaspoons daily
- chlorella - several capsules or tablets daily

A number of products are available specifically formulated for the regeneration of damaged liver tissue. Many of these products consist of a specific combination of herbs. Modified fasting programs have also been determined to be of value in inducing a remission in toxic liver syndromes.

Ideally, each of the protocols should be taken with a large amount of extra virgin olive oil, like a quarter cup. This stimulates bile flow. Follow this recipe: mix 1/4 cup extra virgin olive oil with 1/4 cup high quality or organic vinegar. Add 100 drops of Gene's Greens. Drink half this mixture or the full amount daily, along with the Oregacyn Liver. The Gene's Greens and Oregacyn Liver are potent liver regeneratives.

The Malabsorption Syndrome

Malabsorption is defined as the inability to absorb nutrients from the food into the blood. Millions of Americans suffer from this condition, many unknowingly.

The digestive tract consists of numerous organs, all of which perform their own unique functions for the breakdown of food and absorption of nutrients. These organs include the stomach, small intestine, large intestine, pancreas, and liver. Defective function of any one of these organs can result in malabsorption.

Nutrients are absorbed primarily in the small intestine. This organ contains a delicate lining consisting of billions of microscopic organ systems called *intestinal villi*. These villi control the absorption of nutrients from the intestine into the bloodstream. Deficiency of certain nutrients, notably zinc and folic acid, leads to the destruction of intestinal villi. So can food allergy, especially allergy to legumes and grains.

Food allergy is perhaps the most common cause of malabsorption. A dramatic example is allergy to grains (gluten intolerance), which may lead to wholesale destruction of the intestinal villi. Other primary causes include intestinal parasitic infection, enzyme deficiency, intestinal bacterial flora imbalance, alcoholism, and reduced stomach acid output (hypochlorhydria).

In severe cases malabsorption leads to widespread nutritional deficiencies. The problem may become so extreme that certain individuals develop deficits of virtually every major nutrient. Not surprisingly, a variety of deficiency-induced illnesses, such as osteoporosis, lung disease, chronic fatigue syndrome, fibromyalgia, immune deficiency, emaciation, ulcerative colitis, Crohn's disease, arthritis, anemia, and liver disease, are associated with chronic malabsorption.

MALABSORPTION TEST

Which of these apply to you (each response worth 1 point)?

1. excessive weight loss or gain
2. greasy foul-smelling stools
3. hair loss and/or balding
4. constipation, particularly from eating certain foods
5. chronic diarrhea
6. undigested food in the stool
7. bloating and indigestion after meals unrelieved by antacids
8. foul-smelling intestinal gas
9. belching after meals
10. chronic heartburn
11. premature graying of the hair
12. hangnails
13. ridges on the nails and/or brittle nails
14. dry flaky and/or chapped skin
15. chronic fatigue
16. blood sugar disturbances
17. tendency to develop cavities
18. seborrhea and/or severe dandruff
19. geographic tongue and/or bald spots on the tongue
20. red or inflamed tongue
21. Has your stomach been surgically removed?
22. Has a portion of your intestines been surgically removed?
23. Do you take antacids on a daily basis?
24. Do you take Zantac or Tagamet on a daily basis?
25. Do you consume alcohol on a daily basis?
26. Are you a diabetic, or do you suffer from hypoglycemia?
27. Do you have lactose or milk intolerance?
28. Do you have an active intestinal or stomach ulcer?
29. Do you take laxatives, including mineral and castor oil, on a daily or weekly basis?

30. Do you have a history of celiac disease or gluten intolerance?
31. Do you have liver or pancreatic disease?
32. Do you have cystic fibrosis?
33. Do you have a history of Crohn's disease, ulcerative colitis, or irritable bowel syndrome?
34. Are you undergoing chemotherapy treatments?
35. Do you suffer from systemic skin diseases such as psoriasis, eczema, and dermatitis?
36. Do you have a history of intestinal parasitic infection?
37. Are you anemic?
38. Do you take antibiotics on a daily or weekly basis?

Your Score _____

---

1 to 6 points *Mild malabsorption:* The symptoms of malabsorption are often vague. However, for preventive insurance you should consider undergoing food allergy testing, since the primary cause of malabsorption is food intolerance. In my experience the finest food allergy test available for discovering foods which cause malabsorption is performed by *Nutritional Testing Labs.* The cost is $450.00 for 204 foods or approximately $2.00 per food. For more information call 1-800-243-5242. This test offers a significantly greater degree of accuracy than other allergy tests such as scratch, RAST, and ELISA tests. It is also of value for individuals suffering from asthma, arthritis, lupus, irritable bowel syndrome, and migraine headaches, all of which are due primarily to food allergy reactions. This is a top quality test, far superior to the typical ones ordered by doctors. On a daily basis take folic acid (about 2 mg) and a digestive supplement.

7 to 16 points *Moderate malabsorption:* Follow the aforementioned advice, be sure to chew foods thoroughly. A Food

Intolerance Test is highly needed. Certain condiments stimulate the flow of digestive juices, including hot/tangy spices and vinegar. Add spices regularly to foods. Use vinegar on all salads and add prodigious quantities of spices to your foods. Take 5 mg of folic acid twice daily. Increase the intake of predigested foods such as yogurt, kefir, tempei, and raw honey. Also, take spice extract/enzyme combination, such as Oregacyn Digestive, 2 capsules with every meal. Also take a healthy bacterial supplement, such as Health-Bac, one teaspoon in warm water daily.

17 and above *Severe malabsorption:* Warning—significant nutritional deficiencies are occurring as a result of intestinal malabsorption. It is virtually assured that food allergies are the major culprit, and, thus, food intolerance testing is indicated. Pancreatic insufficiency and gluten intolerance are also likely. If you also scored high on the test for intestinal parasites, this may be the primary cause of the malabsorption. In addition to the previously mentioned advice take the following supplements:

- multiple healthy bacterial supplement (i.e. Health-bac) - one teaspoon twice daily
- Oregacyn Digestive - 3 caps with each meal and an additional 3 one hour after meals
- folic acid - 5 mg twice daily
- zinc - 50 mg daily
- vitamin B-6 - 50 mg daily
- B-complex - 1 tablet daily
- multiple mineral - 2 tablets daily
- Oil of Ginger (North American Herb & Spice) - 5 drops twice daily
- aloe vera juice - 2 ounces twice daily
- chlorella - add packet of granules to each dose of aloe vera juice

Remember, the cure is efficiently achieved only if the cause is determined, whether food allergies, parasitic infection, yeast infection, or pancreatic disease. If the condition fails to improve, see your physician.

Conclusion

The majority of people are deficient in a wide range of nutrients. Incredibly, nutritional deficiency is epidemic throughout the Western world. Such deficiencies greatly compromise body functions. This results in a breakdown in health, ultimately precipitating disease. Through the nutrition test approach the individual determines the precise nutritional imbalances and deficiencies. This is the first step on the journey to better health.

People experience a wide range of symptoms. They may have specific diseases or signs. They may develop an odd or unexplainable symptom/sign: a rash, brittle nails, or some other seemingly unrelated condition. However, they rarely if ever attribute them to something so simple: the deficiency of vitamins, minerals, enzymes, essential fatty acids, amino acids, and more.

To correct these deficiencies a variety of approaches must be taken. The diet must be changed. The intake of all noxious substances must be curtailed. Plus, the appropriate nutritional supplements must be taken. A person must select supplements which are high grade and, which effectively correct the deficiencies. Nutrient-dense foods and food-like supplements are superior to synthetically-based pills. For example, researchers have discovered that synthetic beta carotene possess toxicity unknown for the natural extract. The synthetic type may even crystallize in the retina of the eye, interfering with vision.

While physicians often fail to recognize it diseases may be caused by nutritional imbalances. A variety of dietary changes as well as vitamin/mineral supplements and herbal tonics may prove effective as a cure. The fact is through natural medicine there is hope for a cure.

The first step is to change your diet and lifestyle. Then, take the appropriate nutritional and herbal supplements. There are certain general tonics, which can benefit virtually all. Each section provides specific recommendations based upon an individual's needs.

Always remember that the finest sources for vitamins and minerals are organically grown foods. Thus, the resolution of nutritional deficiency ideally would be accomplished through dietary correction, that is through the consumption of organically produced fruits, vegetables, milk products, grains, and meats. Soup made with organically-raised foods is an excellent way to achieve this; the broth is extremely rich in vitamins and minerals. Additionally, supplement the diet with nutrient-dense foods (see page 300). However, diet alone rarely suffices for resolving severe nutritional deficits. Supplements play a major role here.

The ancillary nutrients, such as antioxidants, enzymes, fatty acids, and coenzymes, may need to be supplemented individually. Everyone living in an industrialized or urban region would benefit from consuming extra vitamin E, beta carotene (vitamin A), and vitamin C besides what is received in the diet. Essential fatty acid deficiency is so common in the United States that routine consumption of a natural fatty acid supplement is indicated. Digestive enzyme deficiency is also exceedingly common. A variety of enzyme supplements are available in the market-place made from both animal and plant sources. Check your health food store for availability. However, if the various aforementioned specialty nutritional products are unavailable in your area, they may be ordered by calling 1-800-243-5242 or in Canada 866-377-7423. For more information check the Web site, Oreganol.com.

Tens of millions of people throughout the globe suffer ill health as a consequence of nutritional deficiencies. Individuals reading this book may be surprised to find themselves among the victims. A greater number of people will fail the tests in this book than those who will pass them. This demonstrates the epidemic nature of nutritional deficiencies.

Currently, nutritional deficiency is equally common in the Western World and the Third World. This was thoroughly proven early in this century, notably by the work of Weston Price, DDS. Price traveled throughout the world, visiting both civilized and primitive societies. His work is immortal, since many of the primitive societies he studied are no longer in existence. Price clearly documented the fact that Americans suffer from a wide range of nutritional deficiencies as well as diseases unheard of in most primitive civilizations. His book, *Physical Degeneration*, makes fascinating reading, complete with photographs, and is available from the Price-Pottenger Nutrition Foundation (see Appendix C).

An individual does not have to develop beriberi or scurvy to have a nutritional deficiency. Virtually all Americans suffer from the consequences of nutrient deficits. Recent surveys show that the average American gets significantly less than the RDA for a variety of nutrients, including vitamins A, C, and B, magnesium, folic acid, riboflavin, pyridoxine, pantothenic acid, chromium, manganese, copper, selenium, and zinc. Plus, Americans consume excessive amounts of low-nutrient foods such as white flour, white rice, white sugar, and margarine. As many as 70% of dietary calories may be derived from such devitalized foodstuffs.

Certain individuals, including many nutritional "authorities", maintain that Americans get all the nutrients they need from their food. These individuals claim that the body's nutritional needs are entirely met as a result of the fact that Americans regularly consume foods from all four food groups such as commercial fruits and vegetables. As such, the "experts" are unwilling to accept the undeniable facts: frozen and canned vegetables and fruits exhibit nutrient losses ranging from 20 to 95%. For instance, these experts are apparently unaware that supermarket citrus fruit is usually gas ripened and that often the fruit contains no measurable amounts of vitamin C. Michael Colgan, Ph.D., proved this at the Rockefeller Institute over a decade ago. Yet, it is not common knowledge that fresh fruit is no longer a top vitamin C source.

334   Nutrition Tests for Better Health

The majority of individuals are unaware of the differences between organic food and commercially grown food. This is also true of the majority of physicians and dieticians. The fact is an organically grown tomato may contain a tenfold or even greater magnesium content than a commercially grown one and that it may contain three times the vitamin C and twice the vitamin A? What's more, organic tomatoes taste better. The point is that the current generation is getting significantly less vitamins and minerals in their food, even in fresh produce, than did people living in the era preceding modern chemical farming. It is easy to understand why people are becoming severely deficient. A reasonable estimate is that people today receive less than one-third the minerals of that of the previous generations prior to 1950. As a result, mineral deficiency is rampant in the USA. Linus Pauling claimed that mineral deficiency is one of the greatest causes of today's diseases.

Food fortification fails to correct the widespread nutritional deficiencies. In fact, this process creates more problems than it solves. Relatively few vitamins are added to foods, and the only foods which are fortified are products containing white flour, refined corn, or white rice (milk products are also vitamin-fortified). What's more, the vitamin/mineral mix added by food processors contains a toxin: inorganic iron. This form of iron binds to and inactivates certain nutrients, notably vitamin E and vitamin C. Thus, inorganic iron is a nutrient robber, not a fortifier. White rice and flour are lacking in dozens of nutrients. What good is accomplished by the addition of a few milligrams of B-vitamins and inorganic iron when dozens of other nutrients are missing? The original food quality cannot be resurrected by such an incomplete approach. In fact, a good rule is that if a food has been fortified, avoid it. Milk products may be an exception, since they are fortified with vitamin D, a nutrient sorely needed by the majority of Americans.

The nutritional tests in this book allow people to determine their precise nutritional deficiencies. Then, the information must be acted upon. If no action is taken, the deficiencies will only deepen with time, and the risks for degenerative diseases will rise correspondingly. On the other hand, if the diet is altered and supplementation is applied, improved health will result.

If you are healthy, use the nutrition tests as a means to fine tune your health, that is upgrade it, so that you may remain healthy for your entire lifetime. Ninety days after beginning a corrective program, repeat those tests on which you scored poorly. This will help in monitoring any improvement. As a result of changing the diet and taking the supplements rapid improvement should be expected. A significant reduction in symptoms, for instance, improving from a severe to a mild category, is a signal that you are "on the right track." Above all, do not procrastinate. No one can afford the prospect of ill health, since it may be difficult for the individual to rebuild his/her health once it has deteriorated.

This is a strategic program based upon precise information: about the individual. Thus, positive results routinely occur. In other words, because this system is scientifically based the results are usually profound.

The health status of the body and mind are inseparable. The fact is our minds are affected by what we eat or fail to eat. The function of the body and mind will improve as a consequence of nutritional revitalization. The result is a greater degree of strength and energy, enhanced beauty, serenity and happiness, and a sharper-thinking mind. These benefits must be expected as a result of improved nutrition.

The brain requires nutrients, and if its nutrition is compromised, a wide range of symptoms may develop: headaches, mental fatigue, memory loss, depression, apathy, anxiety, agitation, anger, mood swings, suicidal thoughts, and even violent behavior. When it is fed poorly and when it is deprived of essential nutrients, the body revolts. The results are: fatigue, pain, digestive disturbances, nerve disorders, and, ultimately, disease.

Ultimately, severe nutritional deficiencies result in a breakdown of the body. In contrast, a solid nutritional program keeps the body vital. No one wants to live his/her later years like an invalid, as so many do today. Nursing homes and mental hospitals are filled to capacity. The occupants uniformly live a poor quality of life. Sadly, their health is so defective that they can no longer care for themselves. Such individuals are grossly deficient in a wide range of nutrients. What's more, when institutionalized, the deficiencies deepen. The fact is the diets in such institutions are unfit for human consumption. As a result, the elderly and/or disabled develop a wide range of nutritional deficiencies, leading both to various symptoms and diseases. Unfortunately, instead of correcting the deficiencies, physicians prescribe drugs, which accelerate nutrient loss and impair the absorption of vitamins and minerals.

Institutionalized patients struggle to survive each day. Most people would rather be dead than to live this way. Hospitalized patients suffer a similar dilemma, that is nutritionally speaking. The same bland empty-nutrient diet is fed to them as well. As a rule, institutionalized food is tasteless, starchy, nutritionally depleted, and overcooked. It is as if bland food is the determinant for how good it is for you. What is the nutritional value of twice overcooked oatmeal, white bread, saltines, pastries, puddings, biscuits, instant potatoes, white rice, gravies, canned fruit, Jello, canned vegetables, extra well-done meats, margarine, muffins, jelly, cane sugar, and 7-Up? It is nil.

Hospital foods violate every rule of sound nutrition. As an example of the extensive nutritional ignorance of the medical profession one of the most noxious of all foodstuffs, deep-fried foods, is still on the menu in all hospitals. Whole grains are an anomaly. Regarding fresh chemical-free fruits and vegetables, they are a rare delicacy. Hospital dieticians plan menus which are constrained by the budget rather than nutritional composition. So it appears they have no understanding of what a nutritionally competent diet is. Nutritional deficiencies in hospitalized patients are rampant. The food not only tastes bad but is bad for you, especially if you are already sick. Therefore, generally, hospitals are not the place to gain wellness.

For those who are in good health the knowledge gained from reading this book can be applied for prevention and for keeping the body and mind fit and strong. Regarding illness the nutritional approach is ideal, because in contrast to drug therapy it treats the cause rather than the symptoms.

Symptoms are the key, that is to determining the cause. A continuous battle with various sicknesses places great stress on the body, even accelerating aging. By systematically analyzing the symptoms, as well as signs, the exact nutritional deficiencies, as well as disease states, are determined.

Many people take an apathetic view of such an effort, that is symptom analysis. This is to their detriment, since symptoms warn of internal disorder, including life-threatening diseases. Even a modest effort at reversing the cause can lead to tremendous results.

Fatigue is not an inevitable consequence of aging nor is memory loss, hunched posture, chronic pain, hearing loss, and wrinkled skin. If the exact nutritional deficiencies can be discovered early enough and aggressively corrected, the aging process can be stalled or even reversed. Thus, it is possible to feel good and look vital despite the acceleration of years.

The diet is simple. Avoid all toxins and processed foods listed in the self-tests. Eat wholesome foods and avoid any foods to which you are allergic. Steer clear of food faddism. Instead, concentrate on the invigorating value of all of the God-given foods: fruits, vegetables, fresh meats, eggs, dairy products, nuts, seeds, and whole grains.

Persistence is the key to nutritional correction. Following the diet temporarily or taking the nutrients for only a few days won't resolve the problem. It took a long time for the individual to get in his/her current condition, and it will take many days, weeks, or months for the full benefits of rehabilitation to be realized. Take your nutritional supplements regularly, preferably two or three times daily. Ideally, emphasize truly natural-based supplements such as crude red grape powder, oil of wild oregano, wild oregano herb, unprocessed royal jelly, crude pumpkinseed oil, and unprocessed brown rice fractions. Don't be confused by marketing glitz. Be sure the supplements are truly natural and are free of any harmful contaminants. The fact that natural vitamins are superior to the synthetic offers proof of a truly mighty, higher being. The Maker of these vitamins causes them to fit perfectly within cells, many of the synthetic types fail to do so. If possible, get natural source vitamin and mineral supplements. These are made by North American Herb & Spice Co.

Anyone can stall the aging process. In order to achieve this it is necessary to religiously follow a nutritious diet. What's more, by making the necessary dietary changes virtually anyone can gain benefits. To achieve optimal health the person must curtail the intake of all stimulants and depressants. All types of processed and chemically-treated foods must be eliminated. There must be a regular intake of whole food supplements. As a result, the individual will achieve the immense benefits of improved nutrition: superior health, improved vitality, enhanced mental powers, increased physical strength, and a fuller, longer and happier life.

Appendix A

Dietary Sources of Nutrients

Top Sources of Vitamin A

alfalfa leaf meal
apricots, dried or raw
arugula
asparagus
beet greens
broccoli
butter
butternut squash
cantaloupe
capers
carrot juice
carrots
chlorella and spirulina
cod liver oil
collards
crab
dandelion greens
egg yolks
endive
escarole
halibut
hot red chili peppers

kale
liver (calf, lamb, beef)
nectarines
oysters
paprika
parsley
parsley juice
peaches, dried or raw
persimmons
pimentos
pumpkin
salmon
sea plasma
spinach
sweet potatoes
Swiss chard
swordfish
tomato juice
turnip greens
watercress
winter squash

Top Sources of Vitamin B-12

catfish
chlorella
clams
cod
crab
eggs
fish eggs (from herring,
cod, or mackerel)
haddock
herring

kidneys
liver (beef or lamb)
mozzarella cheese
oysters (raw)
red meats
salmon
sardines
spirulina
tuna

Top Sources of Vitamin B-6

almonds
bananas
beef or lamb liver
Brazil nuts
brewer's yeast
brown rice
chicken (white meat is best)
fresh peanut butter
fresh sweet corn
halibut
hazelnuts
parsley, dried

peanuts
pecans
rice bran
salmon mackerel
soybean flour
sunflower seeds
torula yeast
tuna
walnuts
wheat germ and bran
whey

Top Sources of Vitamin C

acerola berries
broccoli
cabbage (red)
chili powder
collards
coriander leaf, dried
grapefruit juice
grapefruits
guavas
hot chili peppers
kale
kiwi fruit
lamb's quarters
lemon or lime juice
lemons

mustard greens
orange juice
oranges
papaya
parsley (raw)
red sweet peppers
rose hips
Spanish orange
spinach
strawberries
Swiss chard
tomato juice
turnip and beet greens
watercress

Top Sources of Vitamin D

beef or lamb liver
butter
cheese
cod liver or cod liver oil
cream
egg yolks
fish eggs (roe)

herring
mackerel
salmon
sardines
tuna
whole milk (vitamin D
fortified)

Top Sources of Vitamin E

almond oil
almonds
asparagus
avocado oil
avocados
Brazil nuts
brown rice
cabbage
egg yolks
extra virgin olive oil
fresh peanut butter
hazelnut oil
hazelnuts

organ meats
peanuts
pecans
red meat
safflower oil
salmon and tuna
shrimp and lobster
soy bean oil
spinach
sunflower oil
sweet potatoes
wheat germ (raw)
wheat germ oil

Top Sources of Vitamin K

alfalfa meal
asparagus
beef or lamb liver
beet greens
broccoli
Brussels sprouts
butter
cabbage
cauliflower
cheese

coffee
fresh red meats
green tea
kale
kohlrabi
lettuce
oats
spinach
turnip greens
watercress

Top Sources of PABA

blackstrap molasses
eggs
lecithin
liver

peanuts
soybeans
wheat germ

Top Sources of Thiamine (B-1)

Brazil nuts
brewer's yeast
coriander leaf, dried
oat bran
organ meats
pine nuts (or pinion)
red muscle meats

rice bran
sesame seeds
soybean flour
sunflower seed flour
sunflower seeds
torula yeast
wheat germ

Top Sources of Riboflavin

almonds
brewer's yeast
cheese
eggs
kidney
liver (beef and lamb)

mushrooms (raw)
soybean flour
turnip greens
wheat bran
whey
whole milk (fresh)

Top Sources of Niacin

beef
brewer's yeast
brown rice
chicken
green peas
halibut
instant coffee
lamb
liver and kidney
mackerel
mushrooms
paprika

peanuts or peanut butter
pheasant
quail
rabbit
rice bran
rice polishings
salmon
tomato paste
trout
tuna
turkey
wheat bran and germ

Top Sources of Pantothenic Acid

beans
beef heart
blue cheese
brewer's yeast
brown rice
buckwheat flour
buttermilk
egg yolks
kidney
mushrooms
peanut butter

peanuts
pecans
rice bran
rice polishings
salmon
sesame seeds
soybean flour
tahini
torula yeast
wheat bran
whey

Top Sources of Folic Acid

almonds
avocados
beets and beet tops

mangos
mulberries
oranges

boysenberries
Brie cheese
broccoli
cabbage (raw)
cantaloupe
cauliflower
chicken (dark meat)
cottage cheese
egg yolks
endive (curly or escarole)
fresh peanut butter
kale
liver

organ meats
parsley (raw)
peanuts
pineapple juice
powdered milk
rice bran
rice germ
sour cream
soybean flour
spinach
spinach (raw)
turnip greens
wheat germ and bran

Top Sources of Biotin

almonds
beef
cauliflower
cheese
chicken
chocolate
egg yolk
mushrooms

organ meats
oysters
peanuts or peanut butter
rice polishings
sardines
soybean flour
walnuts
wheat bran and germ

Top Sources of Bioflavonoids

alfalfa leaf powder
apricots
bee propolis
black currants
blackberries
broccoli
buckwheat
cantaloupe
cherries
citrus pulp
citrus rind
elderberries
grapefruit

grapefruit juice
grapes
green peppers
hot red peppers
orange juice
oranges
plums
pure raw vinegar
red onions
strawberries
sweet red peppers
tangerine juice

Top Sources of Calcium

aged cheeses
almonds
blackstrap molasses
basil
caviar
celery seed
dill weed
dried figs
hazelnuts
marjoram, dried
oregano
parmesan cheese
parsley, dried (or parsley juice)
poppy seed

rosemary leaves
sage
salmon
sardines
savory
sour cream
soybean flour
thyme
trout
turnip greens
whey
whole milk
yogurt

Top Sources of Iron

anise seed
apricots, dried
basil
bay leaves
beef
blackstrap molasses
caviar
celery seed
cinnamon
cocoa
coriander leaf, dried
cumin seed
curry powder
dill weed, dried
egg yolks
fenugreek seed
liver

majoram, dried
oregano
oysters
parsley
parsley leaves, dried
prunes
raisins
rice bran
sardines
savoy
soybean flower
spinach
sunflower seed flour
tarragon
thyme
turmeric
wheat bran and germ

Top Sources of Chromium

apple peels
blackstrap molasses
brewer's yeast
cheese

eggs
fresh red meats
liver

Top Sources of Copper

alfalfa meal
almonds
black pepper
blackstrap molasses
Brazil nuts
brewer's yeast
cocoa
dried coconut
green olives

lamb meat
liver (beef, calf or lamb)
lobster
oysters
peanut butter
pecans
soybean flour
walnuts
wheat germ

Top Sources of Selenium

Brazil nuts
butter
chili powder
cider vinegar
cinnamon
clams
crab
eggs
fresh whole grains
garlic

lamb
lobster
mushrooms
nutmeg
oysters
radishes
smelt
Swiss chard
turnips

Top Sources of Magnesium

almonds
basil
beet greens
blackstrap molasses
Brazil nuts
cashews
celery seed
cocoa
coriander leaf, dried
cumin seed
dill weed
fennel seed
marjoram

mustard, dried
oat flour
parsley
poppy seed
rice bran
sage
savory
sesame seed flour (or paste)
soybean flour
spinach (fresh)
tarragon
wheat bran and germ
whole wheat flour

Top Sources of Manganese

blackstrap molasses
blueberries
brewer's yeast
brown rice
carrots
cherries, raw
cloves
ginger
lettuce
lima beans

navy beans
peanuts
raw potatoes
rice bran
rice polishings (Nutri-Sense)
soybean flour
sunflower seeds
turnips
walnuts
whole grains

Top Sources of Phosphorus

almonds
cheese
chicken
cocoa
duck
egg yolks
herring
liver
mackerel
nuts
pheasant
pumpkin seeds

red meat
rice bran
rice polishings (Nutri-Sense)
sardines
soybean flour
squash seeds
sunflower seeds
trout
turkey
wheat germ
whole grain flours

Top Sources of Zinc

alfalfa seeds
basil, dried
beef
caraway seeds
cardamom
celery seeds
cheddar cheese
chervil, dried
crab
egg yolks
lamb
liver
maple syrup

mustard seeds, yellow
onions
oysters (raw)
peanut butter
peanuts
popcorn
poppy seeds
sesame seed flour (or paste)
thyme, ground
torula yeast
turkey (dark meat)
wheat bran and germ

Top Sources of Potassium

apples, dried
apricots, dried
avocados
bananas
basil
beans
blackstrap molasses
cabbage
coriander leaf, dried
dark leafy greens
dates
dill weed, dried
figs
grapefruit juice
guavas
melons
orange juice
paprika

parsley, dried
peaches, dried
peanuts
raisins
red pepper
sardines
seaweed or kelp
soybean flour
spinach, raw
squash (winter)
Swiss chard
tarragon
tomato juice
turkcy
turmeric
veal
whey

Nutrient-Dense Foods
(Super-Rich Food Sources of Vitamins and Minerals)

almonds
avocados
bee pollen
beet and turnip tops
bison meat
Brazil nuts
brown rice
caraway seeds
corn bran and germ
crude raw honey
eggs
fresh vegetable juices
ginger
ground flaxseed
hazelnuts
herring
homemade soups
kefir cheese
lecithin
liver (organ meats)
oat bran

pecans
pepper paste
pine nuts
pistachios
poppy seeds
pumpkin or squash seeds
red hot pepper sauce
rice polishings (Nutri-Sense)
salmon
sardines
Sesame seed paste
sesame seeds
spices
sunflower seeds
watercress
watermelon seeds
wheat bran and germ
wild game
wild rice
yogurt

Appendix B

Recipes

General Nutrition Shake

This applies to all individuals, as it supplies a wide range of the basic natural nutrients everyone needs. This is also an ideal shake to boost nourishment in children as well as teenagers.

3 heaping tablespoons rice polishings (or Nutri-Sense)[1]
3 to 4 tablespoons pine nuts or sunflower seeds
teaspoon Redvital powder
contents of four capsules Flavin-C (for crude natural vitamin C)
contents of four capsules Royal Kick
contents of two capsules ThyroBalance
1 or 2 tablespoons crude raw honey, preferably wild oregano honey
8 ounces yogurt or kefir
frozen berries or other fruit (optional)
water, as needed

Combine all ingredients in blender and blend until smooth. Add water to achieve desired thickness. This recipe is rich in thiamine, other B-vitamins, protein, essential fatty acids, and chromium.

Thiamine Shake

3 heaping tablespoons Nutri-Sense
2 to 3 tablespoons pine nuts
1 tablespoon raw sunflower seeds
1 to 2 tablespoons wild oregano honey
8 ounces yogurt or kefir
fruit (optional)

Combine all ingredients in blender and blend until smooth. Add water to achieve desired thickness. This recipe is rich in thiamine, other B-vitamins, protein, essential fatty acids, and chromium.

Riboflavin Shake

2 tablespoons brewer's yeast
3 heaping tablespoons whey
8 ounces whole milk (goats milk is preferable)
2 tablespoons almonds, blanched

Blend all ingredients in blender until smooth. Add water to achieve desired thickness. This recipe is rich in riboflavin, other B-vitamins, chromium, and protein. Natural strawberry flavoring enhances the taste.

Niacin Shake

3 tablespoons brewer's yeast
4 heaping tablespoons Nutri-Sense
8 to 10 ounces whole milk, water, or orange juice
1/2 cup dehydrated apricots or peaches

Blend all ingredients in blender until smooth. This recipe is rich in niacin, thiamine, riboflavin, and chromium.

Pantothenic Acid Shake

1 tablespoon royal jelly or contents four capsules Royal Kick
3 heaping tablespoons Nutri-Sense
8 ounces milk, juice, or water
2 tablespoons liquid pantothenic acid
2 egg whites (from farm-raised range chickens only; be sure to wash the outside before cracking)

Blend all ingredients in blender until smooth. This recipe is rich in pantothenic acid, niacin, thiamine, and chromium.

Vitamin B-6 Shake

2 heaping tablespoons Nutri-Sense
3 heaping tablespoons whey
3 tablespoons raw hazelnuts and/or sunflower seeds
1 tablespoon liquid vitamin B-6
10 ounces cold water or juice

Blend all ingredients in blender until smooth and serve chilled. This recipe is rich in vitamin B-6, other B-vitamins, vitamin E, chromium, and essential fatty acids.

Biotin Shake

2 tablespoons wheat germ
1 tablespoon cocoa powder
3 tablespoons almonds, blanched
2 heaping tablespoons Nutri-Sense
8 ounces milk
1 tablespoon honey, optional
cold water

Blend all ingredients in blender until smooth. Add cold water to adjust thickness; replace cocoa with fruit if you have a cocoa allergy. This recipe is rich in biotin, other B-vitamins, magnesium, chromium, and iron.

Folic Acid Shake

3 heaping tablespoons rice polishings (or Nutri-Sense)
1/4 cup powdered milk
4 heaping tablespoons soybean flour
1 tablespoon bee pollen
10 ounces cold water or fresh-squeezed orange juice
additional cold water as needed
ripe banana or papaya (optional)

Blend all ingredients in blender to desired thickness. Add water to dilute, if necessary. This recipe is rich in protein, potassium, chromium, vitamin C, folic acid and other B-vitamins.

Folic Acid Tropical Fruit Drink

1/2 mango, peeled
1/4 cup fresh pineapple, cubed
juice of three oranges, freshly-squeezed
1/2 whole avocado (optional), peeled and cubed
1 tablespoon bee pollen (optional)
6 ounces chilled coconut milk (optional)
6 to 8 ounces cold water

Add all ingredients to blender and blend until smooth. This recipe is rich in folic acid, vitamin C, and enzymes.

Folic Acid Vegetable Juice Cocktail

2 bunches parsley
4 beets, raw and peeled
1/2 head cabbage (be sure to remove tough outer leaves)
1 bunch curly endive

Wash the vegetables thoroughly under cold water. Juice in a juicer, discard pulp and serve chilled. This recipe is rich in folic acid, bioflavonoids, vitamin C, and iron.

Chromium Shake

3 or 4 heaping tablespoons rice polishings (or Nutri-Sense)
1 heaping tablespoon brewer's yeast
3 teaspoons blackstrap molasses

1 or 2 cups cow's or goat's milk
cold water

Add all ingredients in blender and blend to desired thickness, adding water to dilute, if necessary. This recipe is extremely rich in chromium as well as magnesium and B-vitamins.

Magnesium Milk Shake

4 heaping tablespoons rice polishings (or Nutri-Sense)
6 or 8 raw Brazil nuts
2 heaping tablespoons soybean flour
1 tablespoon cocoa powder
1 or 2 tablespoons raw honey
ripe banana (optional)
12 ounces milk (or cold water)
additional cold water

Add all ingredients in blender and blend until smooth, mixing additional water to reach desired thickness. This recipe is rich in magnesium, potassium, chromium, protein, niacin, and thiamine.

Magnesium-Rich Spicy Vegetable Juice Cocktail

4 tablespoons fresh dill
2 jalapeno peppers, cored, seeds removed
8 ounces Snappy Tom tomato juice cocktail, spicy V-8, or spicy Very
  Veggie
2 to 4 ounces cold water
1 teaspoon celery seed
bunch of watercress or parsley (optional)

Blend all ingredients in blender until smooth and serve chilled. For extra flavor juice watercress or parsley and add to the drink. This recipe is rich in magnesium, potassium, beta carotene, and vitamin C.

Potassium-Rich Vegetable Juice Cocktail

2 cups fresh coriander leaves (cilantro)
1 bunch parsley
1 head romaine lettuce
1/2 cup chopped red sweet peppers
1 carrot, peeled, optional (for additional sweetness)

Add all ingredients to juice extractor; serve chilled. This recipe is rich in magnesium, potassium, vitamin C, and beta carotene.

Enzymatic Fruit-Sweetened Milk Shake

1 or 2 tablespoon(s) raw bee pollen
1/4 cup strawberries or blueberries
1/4 cup diced fresh pineapple
8 ounces fresh raw milk (goat's milk preferred)
2 tablespoons rice polishings (or Nutri-Sense)
1 or 2 tablespoons pure raw honey
cold water

Add all ingredients to blender and blend until smooth, mixing additional water to desired thickness. Drink immediately. This recipe is rich in enzymes, vitamin C, magnesium, and B-vitamins.

Enzymatic Fruit Splash

3 ripe pomegranates, seeds removed
3 kiwis, peeled
1 large papaya, peeled
1 mango, peeled (optional)
2 or 4 ounces cold-processed aloe vera liquid
cold water

Blend in blender until smooth, adding water to achieve desired thickness. This recipe is rich in enzymes, folic acid, and vitamin C.

Protein/Amino Acid Shake

3 tablespoons soybean flour
1/4 cup powdered milk
1/4 cup sunflower seeds
2 tablespoons bee pollen
12 ounces cold water (or milk)

Add all ingredients to blender and blend until well-mixed, adding extra water if necessary. This recipe is rich in amino acids, B-vitamins, potassium, copper, and vitamin E.

Sea Salt/Sodium Tomato Juice Cocktail

2 teaspoons sea salt, (preferably Celtic salt)
6 ounces tomato juice (unsalted)
juice of three or four ripe tomatoes
Tabasco sauce (optional)
cold water
1 tablespoon capers

Blend all ingredients in blender except capers. Add water to achieve desired thickness. Add capers on top. Serve chilled or over ice. This recipe is rich in sodium, other trace minerals, and vitamin C.

Gingerized Liver Regeneration Drink

1 medium raw ginger root, peeled
1 cup black radish (or daikon radish), peeled and cubed
1 bunch watercress, carefully washed in cold water
1 head romaine lettuce, carefully washed in cold water
1 avocado, peeled (as a source of fat to stimulate bile flow)
cold water

Juice the ginger and vegetables; discard pulp. In a blender add juice and avocado and blend until well mixed; add cold water as needed to achieve desired consistency. This recipe is rich in bioflavonoids, vitamin C, potassium, and vitamin K.

Vitamin C-Fortified Fruit Cocktail

1/4 cup strawberries, preferably fresh and pesticide-free
2 kiwi fruits, peeled
10 ounces fresh squeezed organic grapefruit or orange juice
1/2 teaspoon powdered vitamin C

Blend all ingredients in blender until smooth. This recipe is rich in vitamin C and bioflavonoids.

Vitamin K Vegetable Juice Cocktail

1 bunch spinach or watercress
3 tablespoons powdered alfalfa leaves (not the seeds; they are toxic)
2 cups chopped beet greens (wash well)
1/2 head green cabbage, outer leaves removed

Add all ingredients to a juice extractor. Serve chilled. This recipe is rich in vitamin K, vitamin C, bioflavonoids, and calcium.

Calcium-Rich Vegetable Juice Cocktail

1 cup carrot juice
2 bunches watercress, carefully washed in cold water
1 bunch romaine lettuce, carefully washed in cold water
1 bunch parsley
2 teaspoons of powdered calcium supplement or calcium ascorbate
cold water

354 Nutrition Tests for Better Health

Blend all ingredients in blender, adding water to achieve desired thickness, and serve chilled.

Anti-Aging Vegetable Juice Cocktail

3 medium or large carrots, washed and peeled
1 bunch watercress, carefully washed in cold water
4 turnips, washed and peeled
8 radishes (include tops if fresh—wash thoroughly)

Blend all ingredients in blender, adding water to achieve desired thickness. Serve chilled.

Appendix C

Ordering Information for Books and Nutritional Products

The majority of the unique nutritional products mentioned in this book can be purchased at health food stores. For those which are unavailable order from:

North American Herb & Spice Co.
P. O. Box 4885
Buffalo Grove, Illinois 60089
(800) 243-5242 (847) 473-4700
Fax: (847) 473-4780
www.oreganol.com

Price-Pottenger Nutrition Foundation

This non-profit foundation offers a newsletter and health care provider referral service. The referral service provides the individual with lists by state for locating nutritionally oriented doctors/practitioners. In addition, a number of invaluable nutritional books are available from the Price-Pottenger Nutrition Foundation. A sampling of these books includes:

Nutrition and Physical Degeneration
by Weston Price, D.D.S.
Pottenger's Cats: A Study in Nutrition
by F.M. Pottenger Jr., M.D.
Your Family Tree Connection
by Chris Reading, M.D.

Degeneration-Regeneration
by Melvin Page, D.D.S.
Enzyme Nutrition
by Edward Howell
For Tomorrow's Children: A Manual for Future Parents
by Pre-Conception Care, Inc.
Candida Albicans Yeast-Free Cookbook
by Pat Connoly
The Get Healthy Cookbook
by Bessie Joe Tillman, M.D.
Root Canal Cover-Up Exposed
by George E. Meinig, D.D.S.

The Price-Pottenger Foundation produces a quarterly newsletter/journal. It is packed with invaluable information about the latest findings in the fields of nutrition, preventive medicine, ecology, recipe creation, and organic gardening. Articles by Dr. Ingram, who is an advisory board member, are featured in the journal. Address inquiries to the Price-Pottenger Nutrition Foundation, 2667 Camino Del Rio South, #109, San Diego, CA 92108, or call 1-800-Foods-4-U (1-800-366-3748).

Bibliography

Abraham, A.S., et al. 1987. Magnesium in the prevention of lethal arrhythmias in acute myocardial infarction. *Arch. Intern. Med.* 147:753.

Adams, P.W., et al. 1973. Effect of pyridoxine hydrochloride (vitamin B-6) upon depression associated with oral contraception. *The Lancet* 1:899.

Coggeshall, J.C., Heggers, J.P., Robson, MC., et al. 1985. Biotin status and plasma glucose in diabetics. *Annal. N.Y Acad. Sci.* 447:389.

Collip, P.J., et al. 1975. Pyridoxine treatment of childhood bronchial asthma. *Ann. Allergy.* 35:93.

Collins, ER., and P. Ardt. 1980. Inhibition of C. Albicans by lactobacilli and lactobacillic fermented dairy products. *FEMS Micro. Rev.* (Sept.), 46:343.

Cook, J.D., et al. 1974. Serum ferritin as a measure of iron in normal subjects. *Amer. J. Clin. Nutr.* 27:9681-87.

Cragin, RB. 1962. The use of bioflavonoids in the prevention and treatment of athletic injuries. *Med. Times* 90:529.

Crittinden, P.J. 1948. Studies on the pharmacology of biotin. *Arch. mt. Pharm. Ther.* 76:263.

Curtis, AC., and R.S. Baliner. 1939. The prevention of carotene absorption by liquid petrolatum. *JAMA* 113:1785.

Dakashinamurti, K., and H.N. Bhagavan (eds). 1985. *Biotin.* New York: The New York Academy of Science.

Davis, Adelle. 1965. *Lets Get Well.* New York: Signet.

Davies, S., and A. Stewart. 1987. *Nutritional Medicine.* London: Pan Books.

Dean, R., and K. Cheesman. 1987. Vitamin E protects against free radical damage in lipid environment *Bioc.* Biop. R. 148:1277-82.

DiLuzio, N.R. 1973. Antioxidants, lipid peroxidation, and chemical-induced liver injury. *Fed.* Proc. 32:1875-81.

Diplock, AT. 1980. The role of vitamin E and selenium in the prevention of oxygen-induced tissue damage. In. Selenium in Biology and Medicine, *Proceedings Second International Symposium.* Westport, CT: AVI Publ.

Drake, M.E. 1986. Panic attacks and excessive aspartamine ingestion. *The Lancet* 2:631.

Editor. 1992. Neurologic signs of B-12 deficiency. *Emergency Med.* July, pp. 198-202.

Editors. 1984. *The Complete Book of Vitamins.* Emniaus, PA: Rodale Press.

Ensminger, A.H., et al. 1983. *Foods and Nutrition Encyclopedia.* Vol. 1&2. Clovis, CA: Pergus Press.

Erasmus, U. 1989. *Fats and Oils.* Burnaby, BC: Alive Books.

Fernandes, K.M., and M.A. Shahani. 1987. Therapeutic role of dietary lactobacilli and lactobacillic fermented dairy products. *FEMS Micro. Rev.* 46:343.

Florence, T.M. 1984. Cancer and aging: the free radical connection. bin. *Clin. Nutr. Rev.* 4(1), pp. 6-19.

Folkers, K., and Y. Yamamura (eds). 1986. *Biomedical and Clinical Applications of Coenzyme Q-10.* Bantam Books.

Freedman, A., et al. 1990. Magnesium deficiency-induced cardiomyopathy: protection by vitamin E. *Bioc. Biop. Res. Comm.* 170:1102.

Frolkis, V.V., et al. 1987. Antioxidants as antiarrhythmic drugs. *Cardiology* 74:124.

Frost, D.V, and P.M. Lish. 1975. Selenium in biology. *Ann. Rev. Pharm.* 75:259-84.

Fujisawa, K., Suzuki, H., et al. 1984. Therapeutic effects of liver hydrolysate preparation on chronic hepatitis—a double blind, controlled study. *Asian Med. J.* 26:497-526.

Gabor, M. 1972. Pharmacologic effect of flavonoids on blood vessels. *Angiologica* 9:355.

Gallagher, J.C., et al. 1979. Intestinal calcium absorption and serum vitamin D metabolites in normal subjects and osteoporotic patients. *J. Clin. Invest.* 64:729.

Gibson, G.E., et al. 1988. Reduced activities of thiamine-dependent enzymes in the brains and peripheral tissue of patients with Alzheimer's disease. Arch. *Neuro.* 45:836-40.

Gilliland, S.E., and M.K. Speck. 1977. Antagonistic action of Lactobacillus acidophilus toward intestinal and food-borne pathogens in associative cultures. *J. Food Product.* 40:830.

Gloor, M., and H. Fischer. 1971. Principles of flavonoid therapy. *Fortschr. Med.* 89:1025.

Goldberg, I.K. 1980. L-tyrosine in depression. *The Lancet* 2:364.

Goldman, I.S., and N.E. Kantrowitz. 1982. Cardiomyopathy associated with selenium deficiency. *NEJM* 305:701.

Green, H.N., and E. Mellanby. 1928. Vitamin A as an anti-infective agent. *Br. Med. J.* 20:691.

Greenwood, J. 1965. Optimal vitamin C intake as a factor in the preservation of disc integrity. *Med. Ann. Distr.* Col. 33:274.

Hackney, J.D., et al. 1975. Experimental studies on human health effects of air pollutants. II Ozone. *Arch. Envir. Hlth.* 30:379-84.

Halliwell, B., and J.M.C. Gutteridge. 1984. Lipid peroxidation, oxygen radicals, cell damage, and antioxidant therapy. *The Lancet*, pp. 1396.

Hammar, M., Larson, L, and L. Tegler. 1981. Calcium treatment of leg cramps in pregnancy. *Acta. Obstet. Gynecol. Scand.* 60:345-47.

Haun, R.J. 1992. Indicators of poor nutritional status in older Americans. *Amer. Fain. Phys.* Jan, pp. 219-27.

Havsteen, B. 1983. Flavonoids, a class of natural products of high pharmacological potency. *Biochem. Pharm.* 32:1141.

Heimburger, D., et al. 1987. Improvement in bronchial squamous metaplasia in smoker treated with folate and B-12. *Amer. J. Clin. Nutr.* 45:866.

Hill, M.J., Drasar, B.S., Aries, V., et al. 1971. Bacteria and the etiology of cancer of the large bowel. *The Lancet* 1:95-100.

Hingerty, D. 1957. The role of magnesium in adrenal insufficiency. *Biochem. J.* 66:429-31.

Horrobin, DR. and M.S. Manku. 1983. Essential fatty acids in clinical medicine. *Nutrition and Health* 2:127-34.

Horwitt, M.K. 1980. Relative biological values of D-alpha-tocopheryl acetate and all-rac-A tocopheryl acetate in man. *Amer. J. Clin. Nutr.* 33:1856.

Horwitt, M.K. 1980. Therapeutic use of vitamin E in medicine. *Nutr. Rev.* 38(3).

Ingram, Cass. 1989. *How to Eat Right and Live Longer.* Cedar Rapids, IA: Knowledge House.

Iseri, L.T., et al. 1975. Magnesium deficiency and cardiac disorders. *Amer. J. Med.* 58:837.

Ishiyama, T., et al. 1976. A clinical study of the effect of coenzyme Q on congestive heart failure. *Japan Heart J.* 17:32.

Isselbacher, K.J. 1977. Metabolic and hepatic effect of alcohol. *NEJM* (Mar), 296(11).

Jacobsen, H.N., et al (eds). 1983. *Manual of Clinical Nutrition.* Pleasantville, NJ: Nutrition Publications, Inc.

Johns, DR. 1986. Migraine provoked by aspartame. *NEJM.*

Johnson, F.C. 1979. The antioxidant vitamins. *CRC Crit. Rev. Food Sci. Nutr.* 11:217-309.

Kamm, J.J., Dashman, T., Newark, H., et al. 1977. Inhibition of amine nitrite hepatotoxicity by alpha-tocopherol. *Toxicol. Appl. Pharm.* 41:575-83.

Karkkainen, P., et al. 1986. Alcohol intake correlated with serum trace elements. Alc. *Alcohol* 23:279-82.

Kaul, T.N., Middleton, E., and P.L. Ogra. 1985. Anti-viral effect of flavonoids on human viruses. *J. Med. Viral.* 15:71-9.

Khan, A., et. al. 1990. Insulin potentiating factor and chromium content of selected foods and spices. *Biol. Tr. Elem. Res.* 24:183.

Kligman, A., et al. 1981. Oral vitamin A in acne vulgaris. *mt. J. Derm.* 20:278.

Kok, FJ., et al. 1986. Dietary sodium, calcium, and potassium and blood pressure. *Amer. J. Epid.* 123:1043-48.

Kolata, G. 1982. Heart study produces a surprise result. *Science* 218:31-2.

Kondoh, M., et al. 1984. Effect of sodium saccharin on rate pancreatic enzyme secretion. *J. Nutr. Sci. Vitam.* 30:569.

Krause, M.V., and L.K. Mahan. 1984. *Food, Nutrition, and Diet Therapy.* Philadelphia: W.B. Saunders Co.

Krinsky, N., et al. 1982. Interaction of oxygen and oxy-radicals with carotenoids. *J. Can. Res. Clin. Onco.* 69:205.

Kromhout, D. 1992. Dietary fatty acids, serum cholesterol, and 25-year mortality from coronary heart disease: The Seven Countries Study. *Circulation* 85:864.

Lawson, M., et al. 1987. The effect of dietary fibre on apparent absorption of zinc, copper, iron and manganese in the elderly. *P Nutr. Soc.* 46:53A.

LeGrady, D., et al. 1987. Coffee consumption and mortality in the Chicago Western Electric Company. *Am. J. Epid.* 126:803.

Lesser, M. 1980. *Nutrition and Vitamin Therapy.* New York: Bantam.

Leonart, M.S.S. 1989. Effect of vitamin E on red blood cell preservation. Braz. J. Med. Biol. Res. 22:85-6.

Lindenbaum, J., et al. 1988. Neuropsychiatric disorders caused by cobalamin deficiency in the absence of anemia or macrocytosis. NEJM 318:1720-28.

Littarru, G.P., Ho, L., and K. Folkers. 1972. Deficiency of coenzyme Q-10 in human heart disease. II. internat. J. Vit. Res. 42:413.

Lonsdale, D. 1987. Thiamine and its fat soluble derivatives as therapeutic agents. mt. Gun. Nutr. Rev. 1(3):114-25.

Manson, J., et al. 1992. A prospective study of vitamin C and incidence of coronary heart disease in women. Circulation 85:865.

Massey, L., et al. 1988. Acute effects of dietary caffeine and aspirin on urinary mineral excretion in pre- and postmenopausal women. Nutr. Res. pp. 845-51.

Matz, R. 1993. Magnesium Deficiencies and Therapeutic Uses. Hospital Practice. Apr 30.

McClain, C.J., and L. Su. 1983. Zinc deficiency in the alcoholic: a review. Alcoholism: Clin. and Exper. Res. 7(1).

Middleton, E. 1984. The flavonoids, trends in pharmaceutical science. Science 5:335.

Mock, D., Johnson, S., and R. Holman. 1988. Effects of biotin deficiency on serum fatty acid composition: evidence for abnormalities in humans. J. Nutr. 118:342.

Moses, H.A. 1979. Trace elements: an association with cardiovascular diseases and hypertension. J. Natl Med. Assoc. 71:227-28.

Mussalo-Rauhanuna, H., et al. 1987. Decreased serum selenium and magnesium levels in drunkeness arrestees. Drug Alc. Dep. 20:95.

Niki, E., Tsuchiya, J. Yoshikawa, Y., et al. 1986. Oxidation of lipids. XIII. Anti oxidant activities of alpha-, beta-, gamma-, and delta-tocopherols. Bull. Chem. Soc. Jpn. 59:497-501.

Oelgetz, AW., et al. 1935. The treatment of food allergy and indigestion of pancreatic origin with pancreatic enzymes. Amer. J. Dig. Dis. Nutr. 2:422-426.

Oelgetz, AW., et al. 1939. Pancreatic enzymes and food allergy. Med. Rec. 150:276-279.

Paris, R., and J. Moury. 1964. Effects of diverse flavonoids upon capillary permeability. Ann. Pharm. Frac. 22:489-923.

Perry, H.M. 1978. *Effect of Nutrient Deficiencies in Man: Selenium in Handbook Series in Nutrition and Food*, Sect. E., Vol. III, M. Rechcigl ed., CRC Press.

Peticone, F., et al. 1988. Protective magnesium treatment in ischemic dilated cardiomyopathy (meeting abstract). *J. Am. Col. Nutr.* 7:403.

Prasad, K.N. 1983. Effects of tocopherol on morphological alterations and growth inhibition in melanoma cells in culture. *Cancer Res.* 42:550.

Prasad, K.N. 1984. Nutrition and cancer. In *Yearbook of Nutritional Medicine*. J. Bland. (ed). 1:178-189.

Raloff, J. 1986. Reasons for boning up on manganese. *Science News* (Sept.) 130:199.

Randi, A., et al. 1987. Orally administered vitamin B-6 prolongs the bleeding time and inhibits platelet aggregation in human volunteers. *Thromb. Haem.* 58:176.

Rasad, A.S. 1981. Zinc in growth and development and spectrum of human zinc life. *TAM. Coll. Nutr.* 7:377.

Reed, I.J. 1953. Metabolic functions of thiamine and lipoic acid. *Physical Rev.* 33:544-559.

Reid, IR., and H.K. Ibbertson. 1986. Calcium supplements in the prevention of steroid-induced osteoporosis. *Amer. J. Clin. Nutr.* 44:287-290.

Reiser, S., et al. 1987. Effect of copper intake on blood cholesterol and its lipoprotein distribution in men. *Nutr. Rep. In.* 36:641-649.

Resnik, L. 1987. Interrelation of calcium and magnesium with renin-sodium factors in essential hypertension. *J. Am. Coll. Nutr.* 6:62-63.

Reynolds, E., et al. 1971. Folate metabolism in epileptic and psychiatric patients. *J. Neuro. Neurosurg. Psych.* 34:726.

Riales, R. and M. Albrink. 1981. Effects of chromium chloride supplementation on the glucose tolerance and serum lipids, including HDL, in adult men. *Am. J. Clin. Nutr.* 34:2670-2678.

Rice, S.L., Eiten Miller, R.R., Koehier, P.E. 1976. Biologically active amines in food: a review. *J. Milk. Food Techno.* 39(5):353-358.

Roe, DA. 1983. *Drug-Induced Nutritional Deficiencies*. A.V.I., Westport, CM.

Roe, DA. 1986. Nutritional Assessment of the elderly. *Wid. Rev. Nutr. Diet.* 48:85-113.

Rogers, 5. 1985. Sugar and health. *The Lancet* Feb. 23.

Rosenberg, E., and P. Belew. 1982. Microbial factors in psoriasis. *Arch. Derm.* 118:1434-1444.

Sandine, W.E. 1979. Roles of lactobacillus in the intestinal tract. *Journal of Food Protection* 42:259-262.

Scholar, E., et al. 1988. Effects of diets enriched in cabbage and collards on metastasis of BALB/c mammary carcinoma (meeting abstract). *P Am. Assoc. Ca.* 29:149.

Schrauzer, G.N. (ed.). 1988. *Selenium in Biological Trace Element Research.* Humans Press.

Schrauzer, G.M. and DA. White. 1978. Selenium in human nutrition: dietary intakes and effects of supplementation. *Bioinorganic Chemistry* 8:303-318.

Schrauzer, G.M. 1977 Cancer mortality correlation studies 111. Statistical associations with dietary selenium intakes. *Bioinorganic Chemistry* 7:23.

Schrauzer, G.M. 1976. Selenium and cancer: a review. *Bioinorganic Chemistry* 5:275.

Schroeder, H.A. 1973. *The Trace Elements and Man.* Devin-Adair Co., Old Greenwich, CM.

Schroeder, HA. 1974. *The Poisons Around Us.* Indiana Univ. Press, London.

Seelig, M. 1964. The requirement of magnesium by the normal adult. *Amer. J. Clin. Nutr.* 14:242-290.

Shamberger, R.J. 1976. *Selenium in health and disease. Proc. Symp. Selen. Tell. Envir.* Industrial Health Foundation, Inc., Pittsburg, PA.

Shariff, R., et al. 1988. Vitamin E supplementation in smokers. *Clin. Res.* 36:A770.

Shaw, D.M., et al. 1984. Senile dementia and nutrition (letter to the editor). *Brit. Med. J.* 288:792-793.

Sohler, A, Kruesi, M., Pfeiffer, 1977. Blood lead levels in psychiatric outpatients reduced by zinc and vitamin C. *J. Orthomol. Psy.* 6(3):272-276.

Sommer, A. 1990. Vitamin A status, resistance to infection and childhood mortality. *Ann. NYAcad. Sci.* 587:17.

Stauber, P., et al. 1991. A longitudinal study of the relationship between vitamin A supplementation and plasma retinol, retinyl esters, and liver enzyme activities in a healthy elderly population. *Am. J. Clin. Nutr.* 54:878-883.

Stevens, R., et al. 1988. Body iron stores and the risk of cancer. *Am. J. Gun. Nutr.* 319:1047-1052.

Suda, D., et al. 1986. Inhibition of experimental oral carcinogenesis by topical beta carotene. *Carcinogenesis* 7:711.

Sugiyama, S., Kitazawa, M., Ozawa, K., et al. 1980. Antioxidative effect of coenzyme Q-10. *Experiontia* 36:1002.

Sullivan, JI. 1981. Iron and the sex difference in heart disease risk. *The Lancet* June 13, p. 1239.

Sullivan, JI. 1983. Vegetarianism, ischemic heart disease, and iron (letter to the editor). *Am. J. Gun. Nutr.* 37:882-886.

Swain, A., Dutton, S.P., Truswell, AS. 1985. Salicylates in foods. *J. Amer. Diet.*

Tanaka, K. 1981. New light on biotin deficiency. *N.E.J.M.* 304:839-840.

Tappel, A.L. 1973. Lipid peroxidation damage to cell components. *Fed. Proc.* 32:1870-1874.

Index

A

Acetylcholine, 60
Acidophilus, 109, 203, 206, 301, 302, 322-324
Addison's disease, 49, 50, 158, 287
Additives, 18, 19, 80, 157, 212, 213, 220, 229, 232, 239, 273, 275
Adrenal Failure Syndrome, 5, 286
Adrenal glands, 10, 49, 50, 53, 54, 73, 134, 143, 157, 159, 160, 181, 239, 244, 245, 248, 252, 286-288, 290-294, 297-299, 316
Adrenal insufficiency, 94, 144, 157, 158, 197, 286, 287
Adrenaline, 56, 77, 286
Adverse effects of farm chemicals, 20
Age spots, 274
Alcohol, 12, 25, 34, 37-39, 42-48, 52-54, 62, 65, 66, 69, 72, 77, 78, 87, 91, 101, 104, 117, 121, 131, 132, 133, 143, 146, 162, 165, 166, 178, 180, 184, 193-195, 200, 201, 209, 210, 237, 277, 280, 284, 288, 290, 292, 296, 300, 311-323, 326
Alcoholism, 62, 177, 197, 318, 325
Aldosterone, 94, 157, 159, 160, 287
Alfalfa, 107, 108, 170, 172, 173, 175, 339, 341, 343-346, 353,
Allergies, 51, 123, 148, 151, 161, 234, 244, 288, 328, 329
Aloe vera, 328, 352
Alopecia, 43, 44, 51, 71, 120, 199,

Alzheimer's disease, 14, 24, 126, 130, 144, 187, 200, 214, 222, 238, 240
Amino acids, 4, 10, 22, 29, 168-171, 192-196, 212, 231, 287, 331, 352,
Anemia, 12-14, 42, 62-67, 105, 106, 118-120, 129, 171, 304, 306, 325, 359
Angina pectoris, 132, 181, 183
Antibiotics, 10, 42, 57, 59, 62-64, 67, 70, 71, 76, 85, 107-109, 131, 167, 194, 195, 204, 205, 206, 231, 299, 301, 312, 327
Antibodies, 55, 148
Antioxidants, 29, 100, 148, 199, 222, 258, 264, 265, 276, 277, 319, 332
Anxiety, 35, 38, 46, 51, 55, 56, 60-62, 64, 67, 112, 116-118, 130, 135, 141, 170, 185, 187, 198, 240, 248, 256, 270, 291-295, 335
Appetite, 20, 35, 41, 46, 52, 63, 67, 71, 85, 90, 127, 132, 141, 143, 145, 158, 163, 179, 200, 235, 281, 282, 288, 305
Arthritis, 7, 14, 20, 24, 46, 48, 53, 55, 60, 62, 85, 87, 91, 93, 95, 97, 100, 110, 119, 126, 128, 132-135, 138, 142, 144, 145, 148, 151-155, 173-175, 179, 186, 197, 200, 214, 222, 234, 235, 237-239, 256, 266, 304, 308, 325, 327
Aspirin, 13, 14, 57, 61-65, 74-78, 85, 90, 109, 110, 128, 131, 135, 146, 176, 194, 200, 252
Asthma, 25, 52, 53, 60, 124, 150, 173, 174, 183, 184, 197, 200, 232, 234, 251, 252, 256, 261, 266, 268, 289, 299, 327
Asthmatic, 123, 252, 260, 261

D

Dandruff, 41, 71, 300, 326
Deep-Fried Food, 220, 222
Dehydration, 4, 206-210
Dementia, 13, 38, 46, 48, 94, 135, 200, 309
Depression, 12-14, 20, 32-36, 38, 41, 46, 47, 51, 55, 58-64, 67, 71, 85, 116-118, 128, 130, 131, 135, 145, 167, 170, 185, 186, 198, 240, 244, 248, 251, 252, 256, 257, 270, 281, 289-295, 335,
Dermatitis, 42, 46, 47, 58, 71, 72, 150, 153, 163, 167, 197, 199, 204, 327
Diabetes, 7, 14, 24, 38, 48, 52-55, 60, 71, 72, 87, 90, 91, 94, 115-120, 144, 148, 151, 167, 178, 179, 187, 193, 194, 197, 214, 222, 235-239, 248, 262, 266, 294, 296, 298, 308, 318, 321
Diabetic neuropathy, 56
Diabetic ulcers, 9
Diarrhea, 20, 46, 63, 90, 97, 107, 120, 132, 134, 136, 146, 158, 179, 199, 205, 231, 235, 258, 288, 300, 305, 326
Diverticulitis, 204, 205, 223
Dizziness, 41, 127, 132, 158, 295
Drugs, 11-15, 24, 45, 57, 61, 62, 65, 77, 86, 90, 98, 107, 109-111, 128, 131, 132, 146, 147, 150, 162, 165, 167, 173, 176-178, 184, 189, 191-195, 200, 231, 250, 253, 268, 276, 299, 310, 312-314, 317, 319, 321-323, 336

E

Eczema, 41, 44, 51, 52, 60, 93, 97, 150, 153-155, 174, 179, 185, 197, 199, 204, 205, 234, 276, 301, 327
Edema, 60, 145, 261
EDTA, 19
Electrolytes, 156, 207
Emphysema, 77, 87, 91, 105, 124, 184, 197, 200
Endocrine system, 29
Endometriosis, 167, 248, 268, 301, 315
Enzymes, 4, 9, 19, 22, 29, 70, 88, 119, 137, 162, 168, 171-173, 177, 178, 180, 239, 277, 279, 319, 321, 331, 332, 350, 352
Epilepsy, 56, 58, 60, 61, 98, 132, 186, 191-194
Essential Fatty Acids, 4, 14, 29, 55, 70, 196-202, 207-210, 218, 223, 239, 258, 331, 348, 349
Estrogen, 5, 29, 94, 287, 314-319
Eyes, 41-44, 58, 62, 67, 86, 89, 90, 146, 163, 200, 208, 273-275, 278, 279, 282, 305, 320

F

Fainting spells, 49
Fatigue, 12, 20, 24, 35, 41, 42, 46-53, 58, 63, 67, 77, 78, 85, 100, 116, 120, 124, 127, 131, 142, 145, 158, 167, 170, 179, 183, 185-188, 190-194, 235, 240, 244, 251, 258, 270, 285, 288, 294, 295, 305, 309, 310, 320, 325, 326, 335, 337
Fatty Acids, 4, 14, 18, 22, 29, 55, 70, 141, 188, 196-199, 201, 202, 207-210, 218, 223, 239, 258, 287, 331, 332, 348, 349

Fiber, 74, 223, 226, 229
Fibrocystic breast disease, 101, 105, 269, 315
Fibromyalgia, 24, 60, 174, 325, 368
Fibromyositis, 24, 60, 154, 167, 368
Fingernails, 128, 163, 179, 199, 274, 281, 321
Fish oils, 197
Flu, 24, 90, 150, 161, 163, 205, 232, 244, 248, 251, 256, 276, 304, 309, 310
Fluid retention, 55-58, 160
Fluoride, 19, 207, 283, 284
Folic Acid, 3, 13, 18, 19, 29, 32, 61, 62, 63, 65, 66, 69, 122, 166, 168, 223, 257, 260, 261, 265, 269, 270, 303, 317, 318, 325, 327, 328, 333, 342, 350, 352, top sources 342
Food allergies, 51, 234, 328, 329
Food Dye, 4, 249, 250-252
Food dye toxicity, 251, 25
Food dyes, 18, 19, 25, 76, 83, 178, 248-252
Food Intolerance Test, 327
Fungal infections, 124, 150, 151, 244, 287, 298, 299
Fungus Syndrome, 5, 298, 368, 377

G

Garlic, 149, 195, 196, 262, 278, 279, 302, 304-308, 311-314, 322, 324, 345
Genetic defects, 12
Geographic tongue, 163, 326
Giardiasis, 34
Gilbert's disease, 34, 318
Ginger, 139, 144, 173, 304, 307, 322-324, 328, 346, 347, 353
Ginger root, 304, 307, 322, 353

Gingerized Liver Regeneration Drink, 324, 353
Glutathione, 29, 217-219, 222, 258, 262-266, 277, 279, 319
Goiter, 121-124, 280, 281, 294
Goiter belt, 121, 280, 281
Goitrogens, 126, 284
Gout, 52, 62, 65, 138, 164
Gum disease, 142, 185
Gums, 52, 64, 85, 91, 107, 174, 175, 182, 183, 199, 273

H

Hair, 20, 44, 51, 52, 58, 59, 63, 68, 70-72, 89, 97, 120, 124, 128, 142, 150, 153, 154, 162, 163, 166-168, 171, 179, 197, 199, 274, 276, 281, 282, 289, 316, 320, 326
Hair loss, 20, 51, 59, 70-72, 120, 128, 150, 153, 163, 166-168, 171, 179, 197, 199, 274, 281, 289, 320, 326
Hardening of the arteries, 13, 17, 72, 86, 106, 120, 130, 146, 176, 214, 237, 239, 276, 282
Headaches, 12-14, 19, 46, 51, 60, 112, 128, 132, 146, 158, 167, 186, 198, 208, 232, 234, 244, 251, 256, 258-261, 269, 270, 281, 282, 288, 295, 296, 316, 327, 335
Heart disease, 7, 13-17, 24, 25, 48, 55, 60, 62, 72, 77, 87, 91-94, 100, 105, 106, 117, 118, 126, 132, 133, 136, 146, 148, 152, 155, 181, 190, 193, 194, 197, 204, 214, 222, 227, 229, 235, 237-239, 248, 262-266, 276, 282, 308, 319